Clinical Blood Transfusion

Clinical Blood Transfusion

Clinical Blood Transfusion

L A Kay MB BS MRCP MRCPath
Consultant Haematologist Sunderland Royal Infirmary

E R Huehns MD PhD MRCPath FRCP
Professor of Haematology University College Hospital

Pitman

PITMAN PUBLISHING LIMITED
128 Long Acre, London WC2E 9AN

Associated Companies
Pitman Publishing Pty Ltd, Melbourne
Pitman Publishing New Zealand Ltd, Wellington

Co-published by Urban & Schwarzenberg, Baltimore

First published 1985

British Library Cataloguing in Publication Data
Kay, L.A.
    Clinical blood transfusion.
    1. Blood——Transfusion
    I. Title   II. Huehns, E. R.   III. Series
    615'.65   RM 171

ISBN 0 272 79832 0

Typeset in Linotron 10/12 Galliard, printed and bound
in Great Britain at The Bath Press, Avon

Dedicated to **PFK** and **YAH**

Useful reference books

Mollison, P L (1983)
Blood Transfusion in Clinical Medicine, 7th edition.
Blackwell Scientific Publications,
Oxford

Petz L D and Swisher S N (1981)
Clinical Practice of Blood Transfusion.
Churchill Livingstone,
New York

Race, R R and Sanger, R (1975)
Blood Groups in Man, 6th edn.
Blackwell Scientific Publications,
Oxford

Contents

Preface

A sound understanding of the practice of blood transfusion is necessary in almost all branches of medicine. Although there are a number of excellent and comprehensive, large textbooks on the subject, these are somewhat inaccessible and daunting to many readers not directly involved in the subject.

It is the aim of this book to provide a concise and readily available account of the theory and practice of blood transfusion, while giving insight into future developments. The book should be useful to all those practising medicine, surgery, anaesthetics or haematology, particularly those studying for higher examinations. It should also be useful to laboratory scientists and technicians giving them an understanding of the clinical aspects of the subject they need.

We wish to thank Dr A. Collins, Dr D Perks, Mr G Hedley, Dr S. J. Machin, Dr A. Yardumian and Dr C Singer, for helpful discussions.

1 The development of blood transfusion

The possibility of replacing blood loss by transfusion has been considered for a long time, at least since the 17th century. At that time the description of the circulation of the blood by William Harvey led quickly to the first attempts at blood transfusion (Table 1.1). However,

Table 1.1   History of blood transfusion

1628	De Motu Cordis	William Harvey
1666	Dog to dog	R Lower
1667	Animals to man	J Denis
	Man to man	R Lower
	First haemolytic reaction	J Denis
1678	Transfusion forbidden by the Pope	
1818	Man to man	J Blundell
1840	Correction of haemophilia by fresh blood	J Blundell
1884	Saline blood substitute	W T Bull
1892	Syringe method of direct transfusion	von Zeimssen
1900/1	Discovery of ABO groups	K Landsteiner
1914 to 1917	Citrate/salt/glucose anticoagulant introduced, refrigerated storage	A Hustin, R Lewisohn R Weil, P Rous, P Turner
1917	Plasma separation and transfusion	P Rous
1927	MN groups discovered	K Landsteiner P Levine
1932	First blood bank	Leningrad
1940 onward	Rhesus groups recognized	K Landsteiner, A S Wiener and many others
1941	Haemolytic disease of the newborn described	P Levine, L Burnham and E M Katzin
1943	ACD introduced	J F Loutit, P L Mollison
1945	Antiglobulin test introduced	R R A Coombs, A E Mourant and R R Race
1960 onward	Prevention of haemolytic disease of the newborn	R Finn, C A Clarke and others
1950 onward	Introduction of plastics, cell separators, blood products, hepatitis B screening, etc. by many, many investigators.	

because a large proportion of the population carry naturally occurring blood group antibodies, blood transfusion was not really successful until the ABO blood groups were understood. With hindsight one can see that the early pioneers must have had some success.

Considering the frequency of the ABO blood groups it can be calculated that two-thirds of random single transfusions must have been compatible, and only one-third would have given rise to haemolytic transfusion reactions. Early on, transfusions were used only *in extremis*: many of these patients must have died. It was not until Landsteiner's fundamental work in 1901 that transfusion became established as a routine form of treatment. The main landmarks in the development of transfusion are given in Table 1.1.

Now blood can be selected with considerable accuracy so as to minimize any risk to the recipient. The principles of this selection are.

1 The donor blood must not carry a red cell antigen to which there is an antibody in the recipient.
2 It is also necessary to prevent the production of antibodies to antigens on the transfused red cells, as these could make future transfusions dangerous or cause haemolytic disease of the newborn.
3 Transmission of infection must also be minimized.

The first is achieved by selecting blood of identical ABO group of the patient to avoid the most common naturally occurring antibodies. Rarer antigen (donor) antibody (patient) pairs, so-called incompatibilities are screened for by the cross-match procedure (page 215).

The second is achieved by giving blood which has identical blood groups to the recipient. In practice as there are so many blood group antigens involved, only the common strong antigens, such as the rhesus groups, are routinely tested for. More nearly 'group identical' blood is used only in special circumstances, such as with patients who are liable to receive many transfusions (p. 69) and, more commonly, to avoid incompatabilities because of blood group antibodies present as a result of previous transfusion or pregnancy.

The third is achieved by screening the donors for various diseases and the use of sterile techniques during the processing of blood.

The next development in transfusion was the storage of blood for use at a later date. Initially, during the First World War, citrate and later citrate/dextrose was used. During the Second World War it was found that acid citrate dextrose was better and this became the standard storage anticoagulant for over a quarter of a century. Blood could then be stored for 28 days (later reduced to 21) and this allowed the development of the modern 'off the shelf' supply of blood now accepted as the minimum in any country. More recently better understanding of red cell metabolism has led to the production of storage media which allow blood to be stored routinely at 4°C for up to five weeks. The increasing use of blood transfusion, however, led to the recognition of the risk of transmitting potentially fatal viral infections such as hepatitis B and more recently AIDS.

Originally when transfusion was carried out directly from donor to recipient not only red cells and plasma but also certain clotting factors and viable platelets were transferred, and in this sense these transfusions were better than stored blood for certain patients. An important development in transfusion has been the processing of blood to produce a number of blood products. Transfusion is now not only practised to replace red cells or correct hypovolaemia but also to replace clotting factors, give antibodies, granulocytes and platelets.

These developments have considerably increased the demand for blood and have led to technical advances allowing the harvesting of large amounts of platelets, granulocytes and plasma through the use of cell separators. The limitations of supply and the hazards associated with the use of blood have also given impetus to the search for synthetic blood substitutes, but this development is still in its early stages. It is therefore likely that the demand for blood and its products will continue and increase over the next decade. *Therefore no transfusion of blood or its products should be given without a proper clinical indication. This would not only be wasteful but carries a risk of morbidity or even death for the patient concerned.*

Further reading

Oberman, H A (1981) The History of blood transfusion. In: *Clinical Practice of Blood Transfusion*, Eds Petz, L D, Swisher, S N. Churchill Livingstone, New York.

2 The blood groups

The red cell membrane

The blood group antigens are situated on the surface of the red cell membrane. This membrane gives the red cell its characteristic discoid shape with a diameter of 7.5 μm and maximum thickness of 2.5 μm at the rim and a minimum thickness of 1 μm at the centre; its volume is 85 μm³ with a surface area of 150 μm². The red cell is filled with

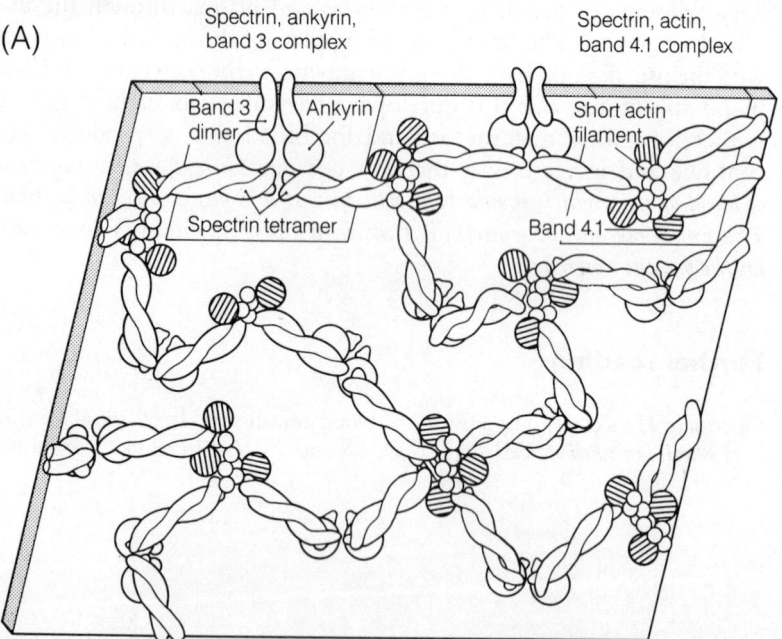

Fig. 2.1 (A) Diagrammatic representation of the network of spectrin dimers and associated proteins forming the cytoskeleton of the red cell. (From Lux, S E (1979) *Nature*, **281,** 426)

haemoglobin and various enzyme systems to prevent haemoglobin denaturation, mainly the glycolytic pathway and related enzymes.

The membrane of the red cell (Fig. 2.1) consists of a lipid bilayer underneath which is a protein network consisting mainly of spectrin molecules; this network is anchored into the lipid bilayer by proteins which penetrate to the outside surface of the red cell. This system is called the red cell cytoskeleton. Besides this there are a number of proteins on the surface of the red cell not connected to the cytoskeleton. This combination of protein network with the lipid bilayer gives the red cell its great ability to deform and maintains the low viscosity of the blood even at high haematocrits, allowing it to pass easily through the capillaries.

It is not clear what maintains the biconcave shape of the red cell. One theory is that the red cell membrane is flexible but not elastic.

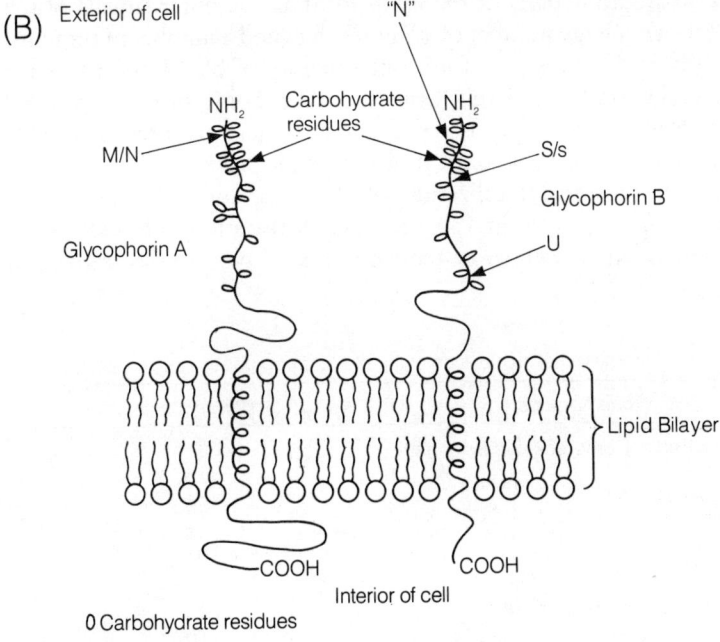

(B) The lipid bilayer of the red cell showing glycophorins A and B. The amino acid sequence buried in the bilayer consists entirely of hydrophobic residues. The carbohydrate residues are diagrammatic. The position of the MN, Ss and U antigenic determinants are indicated by arrows. (Modified from Lux, S E and Glader, B E In: *Haemotology of Infancy and Childhood*. W B Saunders, Philadelphia, 1981, and Anstee, D J (1981) *Seminars in Hematology*, **18**, 22).

Therefore, because it cannot be stretched, the surface area of the cell is constant. The volume of the red cell contents is maintained by the active transport of anions and the consequent movement of water through the cell membrane. In effect the red cell is only partly full and it is this, together with the viscosity of the high concentration of haemoglobin, which gives the cell its biconcave shape. In cells containing less haemoglobin the volume of cell contents falls, although the cell membrane area remains near normal. This results in thin cells with a low volume, but a (near) normal haemoglobin concentration and the appearance of target cells on the blood film.

The high concentration of charged residues on the cell surface causes mutual repulsion of the cells. An electrical potential, the ζ-potential, develops between the negative surface charge and the cell's 'ionic cloud' and this is sufficient to keep the cells apart. The red cell surface consists of the hydrophilic parts of the lipids forming the outer lamella of the lipid bilayer, a large number of sugar residues and a number of proteins. The carbohydrate residues form one category of blood groups, while the proteins on the red cell form the other. Some of these 'protein' blood groups are antigenic *per se*, whilst others are only detectable in the presence of carbohydrate moieties on the protein.

The chromosomal localization of the genes determining various blood groups are given in Table 2.1. The distribution of blood groups and certain other antigen systems on various blood cells is given in Table 3.1.

Table 2.1   Chromosomal localization of the blood group genes

Blood groups	Chromosome
Rhesus, Radin, Dombrock and Scianna	1p
Duffy	1q
Kidd, Colton	2p
MNSs	4q
ABO	9q
Lewis, Secretor (Se)	
Lutheran, Bombay phenotype	19
Xg	Xp
HLA groups (Fig. 4.1)	
A, C, B, D	
Chido, Rogers (complement)	6p
β_2-microglobulin	15q

p: short arm, q: long arm

Carbohydrate determined blood groups
ABO, P, Lewis and Ii

Formation of the carbohydrate antigens

The antigens of the ABO, P, Lewis and Ii blood groups are oligosaccharides mostly (80–90%) attached to protein, but also to membrane fatty acid. The genes for these groups all code for specific glycosyltransferases which attach specific sugar moieties to a simpler oligosaccharide. Thus the A blood group gene gives rise to the A-glycosyl transferase which attaches fucose at just the right position to produce the A antigen. The other transferases act in a similar manner, each leading to the production of its own specific antigenic structure. The different reactions are summarized in Fig. 2.2.

From Fig. 2.2A it can be seen that the ABO and P blood groups are derived from a common precursor. It can also be seen that the P antigen and P_1 antigen are synthesized by separate chains of enzyme reactions and are therefore separate blood groups. The ABH and P_1 antigens are on one common synthetic pathway (dotted in on Fig. 2.2) leading to a second common precursor and finally to the various blood group antigens indicated.

The Lewis blood groups

The Lewis antigens are formed in the plasma from a further common sugar precursor (Fig. 2.2B) and then become attached to the red cell. The secretor gene controls the secretion of the blood group carbohydrates into the plasma. In the formation of the Lewis blood groups the amount of precursor secreted is affected. Secretor negative (sese) individuals secrete only a small amount of precursor which is all converted to Le−a by the relevant transferase. In secretor positive (SeSe or Sese) individuals more precursor (or a slightly different precursor) is produced and some becomes available for the other pathway to form 1H (Fig. 2.2B).

Thus individuals who have the Se gene (secretor positive) form mainly H antigen but also a small amount of Le−a which is always present in the plasma. It has also to be remembered that these reactions do not go to completion and the ABH antigens and Lewis antigens are found together in the plasma and other secretions. The Lewis antigens finally become attached to the red cell membranes. The reason that Le−a is not found on the red cells when both Le−a and Le−b

(A)

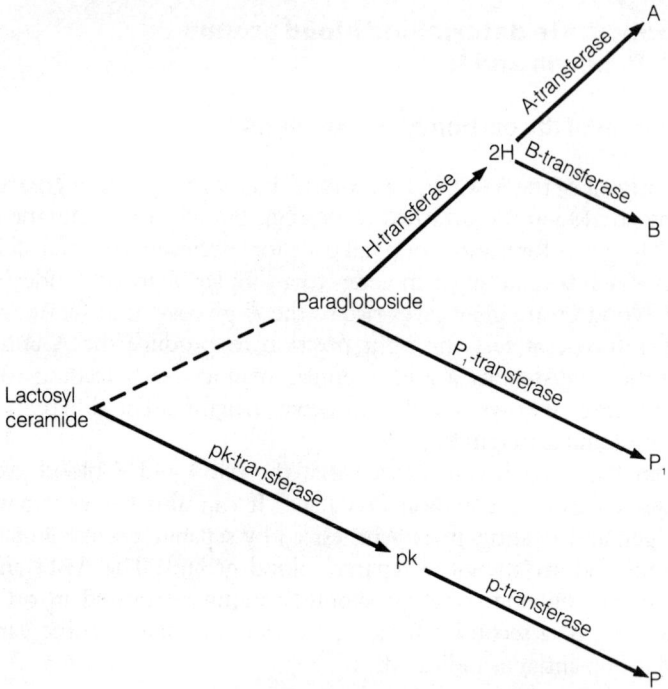

(B)

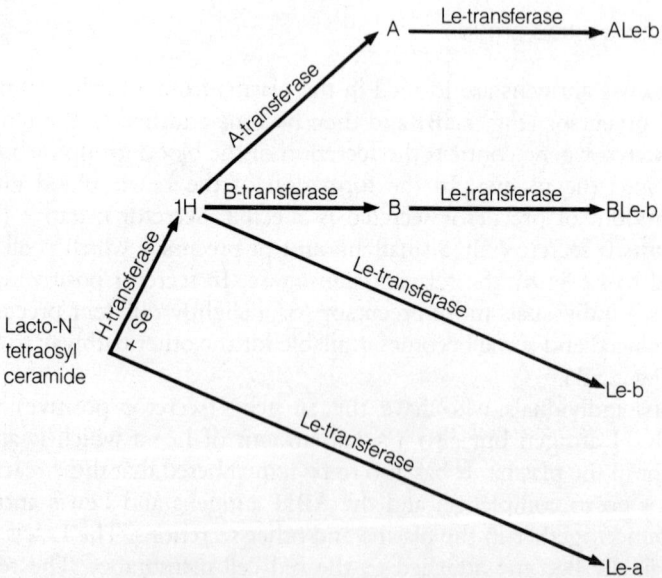

Fig. 2.2 (A) Formation of the ABO, P, and P antigens. (B) Formation of blood group antigens in the plasma.

are found in the plasma is probably because only a small amount of Le−a is made. Both are bound to the same sites on the red cells and the Le−b antigen is taken up preferentially.

The Lewis transferases are poorly developed at birth and only small amounts of the antigens are found on the red cells, thus in cord blood the cells usually group as Le (a−b−). Later in Se (secretor positive) individuals when only small amounts of antigen are produced the cells are Le (a+b+), the amount of Le−b not being sufficient to saturate all the potential binding sites; but by five years there is enough Le−b antigen made to prevent the Le−a antigen binding to the red cells and the adult phenotype Le (a−b+) is found.

The Ii blood group system

In the Ii system the I-transferase converts the i antigen to the I antigen and the relative amounts depend on the amount of this transferase present in the red cells. During fetal life the I-transferase is not synthesized and i is found on the red cells. After birth as more and more I-transferase is made, increasing amounts of I are found on the cells.

The ABO blood group system

The ABO antigens

The ABO blood group antigens found on the red cells are sugar residues synthesized by specific glycosyl transferases. The genes coding for these enzymes are the ABO blood group genes and these are inherited in an autosomal dominant manner. Recent work shows that these are carried on chromosome 9.

Blood group A has two main subgroups—A_1 and A_2. The sugar residues in both these are the same, but they are much closer together in subgroup A_1. It is believed that when the A sugars are close together a new antigen results called A_1. In subgroup A_2 the A sugars are further apart, the A_1 antigen is not present and some of these individuals make anti-A_1. There are no important subgroups of group B. The ABO antigens are present but relatively weak on fetal red cells; they are not found on embryonic (yolk sac) red cells. The frequency of the ABO groups are given in Table 2.2. It can be seen that there are wide differences between various populations.

Table 2.2   The occurrence of various ABO groups in some populations (percentages)

	O	A	B	AB
UK	47	42	8	3
		$A_1 = 34, A_2 = 8$		
South American Indians	100	0	0	0
Chinese	44	26	25	5
West Africans	52	24	21	3
Bengali	22	24	38	16

A, B and H substances on other cells

These antigens are not produced by white cells or platelets and any found have been adsorbed from free antigen in the plasma.

Secretors

About 80% of the population secrete A, B or H substances into the body fluids such as saliva, tears, seminal fluid, sweat, milk, urine, gastric and intestinal secretions, serous effusions, hydroceles, and ovarian cysts and amniotic fluid (of fetal origin). The ABH substance found corresponds to the antigens found on the red cells. The ability to secrete is genetically controlled by the genes Se and se, secretors having the genotype SeSe or Sese and non-secretors (20% of individuals) sese. A, B or H substances are found in all appropriate plasmas but are higher in secretors.

The secretor status also determines the formation of the Lewis blood groups (page 7).

ABO antibodies

'Natural' ABO antibodies

The importance of the ABO blood groups in transfusion is due to the 'natural occurrence' of antibodies. These are believed to form in response to identical antigenic groups found on bacteria in the gut. Therefore all individuals make antibodies to the ABO antigens they do not possess. As everybody carries the H substance the pattern outlined in Table 2.3 is found. In very rare group O individuals a haemolytic antibody to H substance, anti-H, is found. It is because of the presence of these naturally occurring antibodies that ABO identical blood should

Table 2.3 The occurrence of ABO antigens and antibodies

Group (phenotype)	O	A		B	AB	
		A_1	A_2		A_1B	A_2B
Antigens on red cells	None	$A+A_1$	A	B	$A+A_1+B$	$A+B$
Antibodies in serum	anti-A anti-A_1* anti-B anti-'AB'†		anti-B (anti-a_1) 1%	anti-A anti-A_1	none	anti-A_1 25%

* Anti-A_1 reacts with the A_1-antigen, but not with A_2 cells.
† Anti-'AB' has both anti-A and anti-B activity on one molecule. If, for example, A cells are reacted with O serum and the antibody is eluted, then the eluate will agglutinate A cells and, to a lesser extent B cells.

be used for transfusion. These naturally occurring antibodies are mainly IgM, but IgG and IgA are also found. They react best at 4°C and are therefore called cold agglutinins. These antibodies (except IgA) bind complement at 37°C causing lysis of the red cells (page 124). Anti-HI is sometimes found in group A_1 or A_1B individuals but is of no clinical significance.

The ABO antibodies are only weakly present at birth in about 5% of cord bloods. They develop in every person during the first six months of life, and reach a maximum titre at about ten years of age after which the titre falls off slowly. The naturally occurring antibodies are:

Anti-A,* which agglutinates all, A_1 and A_2, group A cells.

Anti-B, which agglutinates all group B cells.

Anti-'AB'. This is found in group O serum. It agglutinates both group A and B cells, but the antibody bound to group A cells will after elution also agglutinate group B cells and vice versa.

Anti-A_1. This agglutinates group A_1 cells but not group A_2 cells. It is found in some group A_2 sera (Table 2.3). It is usually only active in the cold and is then not of clinical significance.

Anti-HI is a cold antibody found in some normal sera and reacts with H and I. It reacts best at 4°C and is found at titres less than 64. It is of no clinical significance. Similar antibodies, anti-AI, anti-BI and anti-PI have also been described and are also of no clinical significance.

* Anti-A is sometimes referred to as α, Anti-B as β and Anti-'AB' as αβ.

Immune ABO antibodies

After ABO incompatible blood transfusions, or injections of appropriate blood group substances (contained in human serum, cryoprecipitate, factor-IX concentrate and some vaccines) the titre of the ABO antibody in the blood rises and some IgG may be formed. These antibodies may also be strongly haemolytic. Blood group O used to be regarded as an universal donor and to some extent this is valid. However, it has to be remembered that the blood contains anti-A + A_1 + B and if any of these are present in high titres they may lyse the recipient's red cells and cause haemolytic transfusion reactions. For this reason group O blood is screened to identify high titre antibodies. During pregnancy the carrying of an 'ABO incompatible' fetus may also immunize the mother and lead to haemolytic disease of the newborn, but this occurs mainly in group O mothers (page 161).

Anti-Hi is an autoantibody which reacts with i and H.

The Lewis blood group system

The Lewis blood group substances are not made in the red cells but absorbed onto the red cells from the plasma as outlined on page 7. There are two Lewis substances, Le−a and Le−b. The precise antigens found in the plasma and on the red cells are affected by the 'secretor' gene and ABO blood group and this results in a complicated pattern of plasma and red cell phenotypes (Table 2.4). It can be seen that if one carries the Lewis (Le) gene and the secretor gene (Se) then the red cell Lewis group will be Le (a−b+), if one carries the Lewis gene (Le) and is secretor negative (sese) then the red cell Lewis group

Table 2.4   The Lewis blood groups

Genotype	Lewis substance in plasma	Red cell Lewis blood group	%
Le, Se	Le−a and Le−b	Le (a−b+)	75
Le, sese	Le−a	Le (a+b−)	20
lele, Se or sese	none	Le (a−b−)	rare

Le denotes the Lewis gene which is dominant, lele—Lewis negative, Se—the secretor gene which is dominant, sese—secretor negative. Se includes the genotypes SeSe and Sese while Le includes the genotypes LeLe and Lele.

will be Le (a+b−) and if one is Lewis negative (lele) then the Lewis group will be Le (a−b−). The antigens on the red cells appear only during the first 15 months of life and during this period the phenotype Le (a+b+) may be found (page 9).

Antibodies of the Lewis system

Anti-Le−a occurs only in about 20% of Le (a−b−) persons. Anti-Le−b is a much rarer and weaker antibody. These antibodies are thought to be naturally occurring. Clinically they are not very important. They do not cause haemolytic disease of the newborn (the antigen is not developed until after birth), but do occasionally cause haemolytic transfusion reactions (see page 206).

The P blood group system

The P blood group system has two antigen types: the P_1 antigen carried only by some individuals, and the P_2 and (related pk) antigen. Their synthesis is described on page 7 and in Fig. 2.2A. These and their related antibodies are given in Table 2.5. None of these antibodies is of clinical significance.

Table 2.5   The P blood group system

| Group | Antigen on the red cells | | Antibodies | Frequency (%) | Notes |
	P_1	P			
P_1	P_1	P	none	75	
P	—	P	anti-P_1 in 60%	25	P_1 antigen absent hence anti-P_1
P_1k (P_1pk)	P_1	pk	anti-P	v. rare	P-antigen absent hence anti-P
pk	—	pk	anti-P_1+P	v. rare	P_1 and P-antigen absent hence anti-P_1+P
p	—	—	anti-P_1+P+pk	v. rare	all P-antigens absent hence anti-P_1+P+pk

The Donath-Landsteiner antibody found in paroxysmal cold haemoglobinuria has the specificity of anti-P and is described on page 131.

The Ii blood group system

The Ii antigens are found on almost all red cells. In cord blood the i antigen is predominant but over the first 18 months of life is replaced by the I antigen as the I-transferase develops. Occasional persons lack the I antigen (i subjects). These individuals carry naturally occurring anti-I. The antigens can also be found in milk, saliva, plasma and on white cells.

Anti-I and anti-i are usually cold agglutinating autoantibodies found in patients with CHAD or following mycoplasma infection or infectious mononucleosis (page 130).

In marrow stress there is increase in 'i' reactivity associated with a decrease of I antigen, and this is a feature of congenital dyserythropoietic anaemia type 2 (CDA2 or HEMPAS).

The rhesus blood group system

The rhesus blood group system is controlled by a number of very closely linked genes leading to the production of the rhesus antigens on the red cells. These genes are carried on chromosome 1. There are three groups of genes: C, D, and E each with a number of alleles; C with c and Cw; D with d and Du as well as other rare forms of weak D; E with e. The presence of these genes leads to the presence of the appropriate antigen on the red cells. All these antigens can be detected by the use of appropriate antibodies, except 'd' as there is no anti-d. There is no antibody reacting specifically with Du or other weak forms of d. Recent work indicates that the D antigen is a protein and presumably the other rhesus antigens are also proteins. It is not known yet whether there is more than one rhesus protein or whether single amino acid differences are responsible for the different antigenic specificities.

As the genes controlling the formation of the CDE antigens are very closely linked they are inherited together and certain combinations are found more commonly than others. To overcome the clumsiness of the CDE notation those who 'live' blood groups use a shorthand devised by Wiener (see Table 2.6). In this book only the CDE notation will be used. When rhesus groups are reported on patients rhesus positive means D antigen positive (DD or Dd) and rhesus negative means D negative (dd). However, in the labelling of donor blood only CDE negative (cde/cde) blood is labelled rhesus negative (in this instance

Table 2.6   Rhesus group nomenclature

	Fisher–Race	Shorthand
	CDe	R^1
	cDE	R^2
	CDE	R^z
	cDe	R^o
	C^{w}De	R^{1w}
	cde	r
	Cde	r'
	cdE	r''
	CdE	r^y

D negative (dd) occurring with the antigen C or E would be labelled as rhesus positive). This has important advantages in blood transfusion as the antibodies to C, D and E often occur in combination (page 18).* In this book rhesus positive means D-positive (DD or Dd) and rhesus negative means D-negative (dd).

Rhesus blood group genotyping

As there is no antibody to the d antigen its presence can only be inferred by failure to react with anti-D and therefore only dd can be detected. Dd can only be inferred from family studies. Using anti-C, c, D, E, e the results are expressed as follows: CcDEe reaction with all five antisera, CCDEe no reaction with anti-c and so on. From these the most probable genotype can be assigned using the known frequencies in the ethnic group of the person being tested. For example an English white person with the phenotype CcDee probably has the genotype CDe/cde (R_1r) but there are other possibilities (Table 2.7). The determination of the D genotype (DD or Dd) is of clinical importance in relation to haemolytic disease of the newborn. If a woman has anti-D in her plasma and her husband is a DD homozygote, then all their children will be affected by rhesus haemolytic disease of the newborn, whereas if he is heterozygous Dd, only 50% of their children will be affected (see page 155).

Subgroups of the D antigen: Du

The Du antigen is similar to the D antigen but lacks some of its reactions, in that it is detected by some anti-D sera but not by others.

* In some centres Cde/cde (r'r) and cdE/cde (r''r) are issued labelled Rh negative, but the genotype is also stated on the pack.

Table 2.7   Determination of rhesus genotype from reaction with anti-C, anti-D, anti-E, anti-c and anti-e from frequencies in Caucasians. The possible genotypes listed account for over 99.5% of the population

C	D	E	c	e	Possible genotype		Frequency (%)
+	+	+	+	+	CDe/cDE	(R^1R^2)	12
					CDe/cdE	(R^1r'')	1
					cDE/Cde	(R^2r')	0.3
					CDE/cde	(R^2r)	0.2
O	+	+	+	+	cDE/cde	(R^2r)	11
					cDE/cDe	(R^2R^0)	0.7
O	+	O	+	+	cDe/cde	(R^0r)	2
+	+	O	+	+	CDe/cde	(R^1r)	33
					CDe/cDe	(R^1R^0)	2
+	+	O	O	+	CDe/CDe	(R^1R^1)	18
					CDe/Cde	(R^1r^y)	0.8
+	+	+	O	+	CDE/CDe	(R^2R^1)	0.2
O	+	+	+	O	cDE/cDE	(R^2R^2)	2
					cDE/cdE	(R^2r'')	0.3
O	O	O	+	+	cde/cde	(rr)	15
O	O	+	+	+	cdE/cde	$(r''r)$	1
+	O	O	+	+	Cde/cde	$(r'r)$	0.8

In practice individuals who are negative with saline anti-D but react when the indirect antiglobulin test or sensitive enzyme reactions are used are classified as DU. Very rare individuals are classified as rhesus positive by all antisera, but their variant nature only becomes apparent when anti-D forms unexpectedly. The Du antigen is rare in whites but occurs more frequently in blacks (Table 2.8).

Although Du is a weak antigen, Du positive red cells can be destroyed by anti-D and can be involved in haemolytic transfusion reactions and haemolytic disease of the newborn. They can also immunize rhesus negative (dd) individuals. For this reason it is usual to classify Du positive blood donors as rhesus (D) positive. In recipients, if the Du antigen is missed, the cells will be classified as rhesus negative (dd) and no harm will result as they will receive rhesus negative blood; if they are classified as rhesus (D) positive anti-D will very rarely be formed if the patient is transfused with rhesus (D) positive blood or during pregnancy.

Other rhesus antigens

The antigen G is an epitope occurring in individuals carrying C or

Table 2.8 Variation in blood group frequencies between populations

	Chinese (%)	Europeans (%)	West Africans (%)
Rh D	100	84	95
Du	—	<1	7
cde/cde (rr)*	0	16	5
K	0	9	<1
Jsª	0	0	20
Fyª	99	65	20

It can be seen that there is gross variation in the occurrence of blood groups between populations and this applies to all other blood group antigens. See Mourant, A E, Kopec, A C and Domaniewska-Sobczec, K (1976), *The Distribution of Human Blood Groups and Other Polymorphisms, 2nd Edn.*, Oxford University Press.
* cde/cde does not occur in Japanese or North American Indians. In Indians it amounts to 8%.

E. C^G is a weak form of C and C^w an antigen associated with C or c occurring in 2% of Caucasians. Ce is an epitope of C and e antigens, only produced when C and e are inherited in *cis*; similarly ce (f) is an epitope found when c and e are inherited together in *cis*. The occurrence of such epitopes suggests that c and e are not separate proteins. V (ce^s) is an antigen found in about 35% of West Africans. There are also rare red cells which lack some of the rhesus antigens: –D– determines the D antigen without any C, c, E or e antigen being present. Homozygotes for this antigen have increased number of D antigen sites. Rh-null cells have no detectable rhesus antigens. These cells may have spherocytosis and haemolysis.

Antibodies to the rhesus antigens

Naturally occurring, IgM, antibodies to the rhesus antigens are rare and are weak, they are not of clinical importance. Immune antibodies to all the rhesus antigens except d have been described. These are mostly IgG, subclass 1 and 3 are the most common but 2 and 4 also occur and, although they react with the appropriate cells, they do not agglutinate the cells. IgM antibodies are rarer and are always accompanied by IgG. IgA antibodies also occur, but only in hyperimmune individuals.

The strongest rhesus antigen is D and 80% of the D-negative (dd) population will form antibodies if stimulated by about 200 ml of blood. The 20% who do not form antibodies are called non-responders. With small amounts of blood, 0.5–1 ml, only about 20–50% will make anti-bodies. Although D is the strongest antigen it is no longer the most common antibody formed. This is because of the care that is taken always to give rhesus negative (cde/cde) blood to rhesus negative individuals, as well as the prevention of rhesus immunization during pregnancy. Anti-C and anti-E are mainly found together with anti-D and are now also less frequent, and anti-c is now the most common with anti-e second.

There are also antibodies which apparently recognize common epitopes on C and D called anti-G. This antibody will recognize both C and D together and separately but, in contrast to the mixture anti-C + anti-D, is completely absorbed by either C+ only or D+ only cells. Anti-C^w may be formed by C-positive, C^w-negative individuals.

All the antibodies of the rhesus system have caused haemolytic transfusion reactions and haemolytic disease of the newborn.

The LW blood group system

The original animal anti-Rh made by Landsteiner and Wiener differs from anti-Rh (anti-D) defining a separate system called LW. Antigens LW^a and LW^b have been described. These are strongly expressed on Rh(D)+ cells. The LW system is not of clinical significance .

The Kell blood group system

The Kell antigens are thought to be red cell membrane proteins. There are two main antigens K and k determined by the corresponding genes. The genes are autosomally inherited, but the chromosome involved has not yet been identified. The gene for k is very common while that for K is relatively rare, thus Kell negative (kk) (Cellano) comprises 91% of the population while Kell positive (Kk 9% and KK 0.2%) amount to 9%.

Antibodies of the Kell blood group system

Naturally occurring antibodies to the Kell antigens are extremely rare, but immune antibodies are the most common and clinically the most important outside the ABO and rhesus systems. The most common antibody found is anti-K formed as a result of transfusing Kell positive (KK or Kk) blood to Kell negative (kk) individuals or due to incompatible pregnancy. However, the Kell antigens are approximately 10 times less antigenic than the rhesus D antigen and sensitization occurs only in about 1 in a 100 transfusions. Sensitization by pregnancy occurs even less frequently; about 1 per 1,000 or 2,000 births. Anti-k (anti-Cellano) is of course extremely rare as the KK genotype occurs in only 2% of the population.

The Kell antibodies are almost all IgG (subclass IgG1) and are best detected by the indirect antiglobulin test (page 209).

The clinical significance of the Kell blood group system

The Kell antibodies, anti-K and anti-k (as well as the much rarer antibodies, anti-Kpa, anti-Kpb, anti-Jsa, anti-Jsb) can cause severe haemolytic transfusion reactions and severe haemolytic disease of the newborn. Occasionally autoimmune haemolytic anaemia may involve antibodies of the Kell system.

Some individuals have diminished amounts of Kx (the precursor substance of the Kell antigens which appears to be controlled by the X chromosome) on the red cells or white cells. This was thought to be associated with one form of X-linked chronic granulomatous disease. If only the red cells are affected, then there may be acanthocytosis and haemolytic anaemia.

The Duffy (Fy) blood group system

The Duffy (Fy) antigens are proteins on the surface of red cells, and are controlled by genes on chromosome 1. There are two common antigens Fy (a+) and Fy (b+), 66% of the population are Fy (a+) (genotype Fya/Fya 33%, Fya/Fyb 33%) the rest, 34%, are Fy (b+) (Fyb/Fyb). As the antigens are destroyed by proteolytic enzymes they are best detected by the indirect antiglobulin test.

Anti-Fya is quite rare and anti-Fyb is even rarer. Antibodies to the other Duffy antigens (Fy3, 4, 5) have only occurred occasionally. These immune antibodies are all IgG, often bind complement and can cause haemolytic disease of the newborn and haemolytic transfusion reactions.

The Kidd (Jk) blood group system

There are two Kidd antigens, Jk^a and Jk^b, controlled by genes on chromsome 2. In the population 26% are Jk (a+b−), 50% Jk (a+b+) and 24% Jk (a−b+). Rarely Jk (a−b−) cells are found in Indonesians, Chinese and South American Indians. This genotype is associated with an ill-defined red cell abnormality.

Anti-Jk^a and Jk^b have been described and are usually IgG and bind complement. They occur as a result of sensitization by blood transfusion or pregnancy. They are best detected by the indirect antiglobulin test. Clinically the Kidd antibodies can cause severe delayed haemolytic transfusion reactions. The antibodies are also a very rare cause of haemolytic disease of the newborn. Occasionally they may be found in autoimmune haemolytic anaemias. Anti-Jk (a+b) (inseparable) (or anti-Jk3) is found rarely in Jk (a−b−) individuals and is usually IgG.

The MNSs blood group system

The M and N antigens are products of two allelic genes, while the production of the S and s antigens is controlled by a linked locus, both on chromosome 4.

The structure of the MNSs antigens

The MNSs antigens are found on the glycophorins or sialoglycoproteins on the surface of the red cell membrane. These form some of the PAS positive bands detected on SDS-PAG electrophoresis of the red cell membrane.

The M/N blood groups differ by two amino acid substitutions in glycophorin A, but need the adjacent sialic acid containing carbohydrate sidechains and the free N-terminal amino group for antigenicity (Fig. 2.3).

Glycophorin B carries the Ss antigens (Fig. 2.3) and these are determined by a single amino acid difference. The N-terminal end of this protein is identical to that of glycophorin A determining N antigen activity. This accounts for the observation that homozygotes for M (MM) always have some N activity. Several other antigens are found on these proteins including U (Fig. 2.1), which can stimulate strong antibody formation in rare U-negative individuals.

Several of the MNSs variants can also be explained on a structural

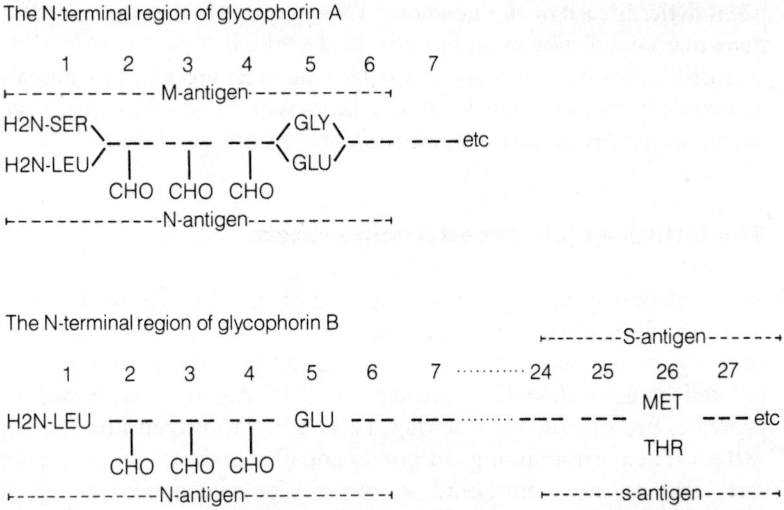

The N-terminal region of glycophorin A

The N-terminal region of glycophorin B

Fig. 2.3 The N terminal regions of the glycophorins A and B. The M antigen differs from the N antigen by amino acid substitutions at positions 1 and 5. The S antigen differs from the s antigen by one amino acid substitution at position 26. Note the N antigen on glycophorin B.

basis. The antigens Mc and Mg are single amino acid substitutions at the MN antigen site. Absence of various glycophorins give rise to certain red cell types (absent a-chain to En (a−b−), absent a− and d−chains to the MkMk genotype, absent d-chains to the S−s− genotype). It is interesting that these individuals are all normal and have increased sialic acids on the other red cell surface proteins. The so-called Miltenberger variants are abnormal hybrids of glycophorins A and B.

Antibodies to the MNSs antigens

Anti-M is a rare antibody usually IgM but may be IgG, it can very rarely cause haemolytic transfusion reactions and haemolytic disease of the newborn. Anti-N, which is rarer than anti-M, has only caused such reactions in very few patients and these have been mild. Occasionally auto-anti-N is found and has caused autoimmune haemolytic anaemia. Anti-N is formed in some patients on renal dialysis, so-called anti-Nf; the clinical significance of this antibody, if any, is unclear.

Anti-S, anti-s and anti-U (more common in blacks) are rare antibodies which can cause both severe haemolytic transfusion reactions and severe haemolytic disease of the newborn. U-negative cells are very rare and there may be difficulty in finding compatible blood.

Anti-M, anti-N, anti-S and anti-s have all been produced in animals and recently mouse monoclonal antibodies with these specificities have been produced which are suitable for blood grouping.

The Lutheran (Lu) blood group system

The Lutheran system antigens are Lua, Lub and Lu (i.e. neither Lua or Lub). Individuals can have the genotype Lu (a−b+) 92%, Lu (a+b+) 8% or rarely Lu (a+b−) or Lu (a−b−). These antigens are red cell gangliosides. They are destroyed by digestion with various proteases presumably because they are attached to proteins on the cell surface. The corresponding antibodies anti-Lua and anti-Lub are quite rare. They are weak antibodies *in vivo*, but have been associated with delayed transfusion reactions and mild haemolytic disease of the newborn.

Other blood group systems

Some of the rare blood groups are listed in Table 2.9. The Xg blood groups are of interest because the genes are carried on the X chromosome and are used in investigating linkage and inheritance of X-linked disorders. They are of no other clinical importance.

The HLA antigens are weakly expressed on red cells mainly on reticulocytes (page 35).

Blood groups in disease

Malaria

Red cells with the Duffy type Fy (a−b−) are resistant to invasion by the merozoite of *Plasmodium vivax*, which can only penetrate Fy (a+) or Fy (b+) red cells. Thus the Fy (a−b−) type is more common in blacks. En (a−) red cells are resistant to invasion by *P. falciparum* as the glycophorins A and B are needed by this parasite for invasion to occur. Wr (b−) red cells are also resistant to invasion by *Plasmodium falciparum*.

Table 2.9   Other blood group systems

Antigen	Occurrence	Notes
Diego		
Di (a)	35% of American Indians are Di	antibodies are haemolytic
Di (b)	(a+), anti-Di (b) made by Di	
	(a+) homozygotes, all Caucasians are Di (b+)	
Dombrock		
Do (a)	Do (a+) 66%	
Do (b)	Do (b+) 82%	
Scianna		
Sc1 (Sm)	Sc1+ >99%	
Sc2 (Ba(a))	Sc2+ <1%	
Colton		
Co (a)	Co (a+) 99.8%	
Co (b)	Co (b+) 9%	Have caused severe HDN
Sd		
Sd (a)	Sd (a+) 91%	Sd (a) is found in the kidney and in the Tamm-Horsfall glycoprotein in urine
Cad		Cad is a low frequency antigen associated with polyagglutination
Vel	high frequency (>99.9%) antigen	antibodies associated with haemolysis
Gerbich (Ge)	high frequency (>99.9%) antigen	some phenotypes associated with elliptocytosis
Gregory (Gy)	high frequency (>99.9%) antigen	
Holley (Hy)	high frequency (>99.9%) antigen	
Lan	high frequency (>99.9%) antigen	
Jr (a+)	high frequency (>99.9%) antigen	antibodies associated with haemolysis
Swann (Sw(a))	rare antigen <1:6,000	the antibody has been found in AIHA
Chido (Ch)		determinants on C4 component (C4d) of complement
Rogers (Rg)		

Rhesus null is associated with stomatocytosis and haemolysis.

The Leach phenotype of the Gerbich system is associated with elliptocytosis.

Kx is a precursor of the Kell antigens and is present on white cells. Its production is controlled by the X chromosome. In chronic granulomatous disease Kx is absent from the white cells in some cases. If it is absent from the red cells, McLeod's syndrome results in which a high serum creatine phosphokinase and muscle fibre changes are found.

In *acute leukaemia* there may be weakening of the blood group antigens A, B and I. Diseases of large bowel may cause the addition of B-like substance onto the red cells, probably of bacterial origin. In dyserythropoiesis, megaloblastic and sideroblastic anaemia there is often partial reversion of I to i. In some myeloproliferative disorders there may be changes in the Rh antigens. Various other unexplained associations have been described. Group A individuals have a 20% greater chance of developing cancer of the stomach than group O persons. Group O people have a 20% greater chance of suffering from duodenal ulcers. Secretors also have a greater chance of developing duodenal ulcers.

Development of the red cell antigens

The *embryonic red cells*, the large (20–25 μm) nucleated cells found during the first two months of development express the rhesus, Kell and Duffy antigens but not the ABO antigens.

Fetal red cells express all the antigens of adult cells except I, Lewis and Sd because the appropriate transferases do not appear until near birth. The ABO, P and Lutheran antigens are weak at birth. The ABO antibodies only appear during the first six months of life.

Paternity testing and identifying blood stains

In medicolegal practice blood groups have been used extensively in paternity testing and for identifying blood stains. In attempting to establish whether a blood stain belongs to a certain individual, the groups of that individual are compared with the groups of the suspect blood. The finding of a blood group antigen difference between the two samples establishes non-identity. However, if both samples have the same ABO blood group, then the blood may have come from the same person. The frequency of the blood group tested is important. If it is group A, then as 42% of random bloods are group A, there is a reasonable chance that it has come from another individual. If it is group B (8.5% are group B in the population), then it is more likely to have come from the same person. However, group B is more common in certain ethnic groups and any assessment must take this into account. If further blood groups can be compared, then the likelihood of identity increases according to the frequency of each group tested and the number of groups examined. As an approximation, the probability of samples being from the same person is the product of the frequencies in the relevant population of each group tested. As only small samples are available for testing, the identities of the bloods can often only be established at a low level of probability. Blood group substances and secretor status are also used in the identification of semen and saliva.

Whether twins are identical (monozygotic) or not can also be established in this way and may be of some importance in bone marrow transplantation as syngeneic (from an identical twin) marrow does not cause GVHD and the management is therefore simpler (page 166).

The occurrence in the child of an 'unexpected' group (not found in the mother or possible father) group would exclude paternity. In this connection the rare occurrence of cis-AB is important. In this the ABO gene coding for the ABO transferase is duplicated. Thus both the A and the B transferase genes can occur on the same chromosome and are then passed on together. If this is a possibility, it can usually be ruled out by studies of the grandparents.

Further information on parentage can be obtained by examining the polymorphic red cell enzyme systems, as well as white cell, serum and HLA types. The HLA system with its many alleles is particularly informative. The more recently delineated DNA polymorphisms may also be useful in future. Usually the probability of a particular man being the father can either be excluded or established with a high degree of certainty.

Further reading

Lux, S E (1979) Dissecting the red cell membrane skeleton. *Nature*, **281**, 426.

Lux, S E, Glader, B E (1981) Disorders of the red cell membrane. In: *Hematology of Infancy and Childhood*, Eds. Nathan, D G and Oski, F A. W B Saunders Co, Philadelphia, p. 456.

Race, R R, Sanger, R (1975) *Blood Groups in Man, 6th Edn*. Blackwell Scientific Publications, Oxford.

Anstree, D J (1981) Blood group MNSs-active sialoglycoproteins. *Seminars in Hematology*, **18**, 13.

Hakomori, Sen-itoroh (1981) Blood group ABH and Ii antigens of human erythrocytes: Chemistry, polymorphism and developmental change. *Seminars in Hematology*, **18**, 39.

Marcus, D M, Kundu, S K, Suzuki, A (1981) The P blood group system; recent progress in immunochemistry and genetics. *Seminars in Hematology*, **18**, 63.

Tippett, P (1984) Genetics of the human red cell surface. In: *Genetic Analysis of the Cell Surface, (Receptors and Recognition, Series B, Volume 16)*, Ed. Goodfellow, P. Chapman and Hall, London.

Mourant, A E, Kopec, A C, Domaniewska-Sobczak, K (1976) *The Distribution of Human Blood Groups and other Biochemical Polymorphisms*, 2nd Edn. Oxford University Press.

Mourant, A E, Kopec A C, Domaniewska-Sobczak, K (1978) *Blood Groups and Diseases. A Study of Associations of Diseases with Blood Groups and other Polymorphisms*. Oxford University Press.

3 Leucocyte and platelet specific antigens

In the same way that the red cells have specific antigens, the blood groups, the white cells and platelets have their own specific antigens. These antigen systems are important in transfusion because the corresponding antibodies are produced in some individuals. These can cause non-haemolytic, febrile transfusion reactions and shorten *in-vivo* survival.

Granulocyte specific antigen systems

Granulocytes carry ABO and some other blood group antigens but these are probably adsorbed. They express HLA class I determinants weakly in comparison with lymphocytes, and it is uncertain whether these are passively acquired from plasma in the same way that platelet HLA antigens are. Table 3.1 shows the distribution of the major antigen

Table 3.1   The distribution of membrane antigen systems on various blood cells

Antigen	ABO	MNSsU	Ii	Rh	HLA Cl.I	HLA Cl.II
Red cells	+	+	+	+	(+)	0
Platelets	(+)	?	0	0	(+)	0
Granulocytes	+	U only	+	0	+	0
T Lymphocytes	+	?	+	0	+	*
B Lymphocytes	+	?	+	0	+	+

Key: + antigen expressed
(+) antigen expressed weakly
  * antigen expressed only when activated
  0 antigen not expressed
  ? not known

systems on various blood cells. Granulocyte specific antigens are found only on granulocytes and are shown in Table 3.2.

Table 3.2   Granulocyte specific antigens

Antigen	Frequency (%)
NA1	54
NA2	93
NB1	92
NC1	96
ND1	98.5
NE1	23
9a	63

Granulocyte antigens can be detected by coating the cells with known, specific antibody. This can be detected by leukoagglutination, but false positives may occur due to the tendency of granulocytes to clump spontaneously. Coating of the cells can also be detected by the uptake of a fluorescent 'second layer' antibody, or by the consumption of added anti-human globulin. Again false positives may occur due to the non-specific absorption of immunoglobulins from the plasma. 'Granulocyte toxicity assays' rely on the fact that added complement when fixed by specifically attached antibody results in cell death. Using these techniques several granulocyte specific antigen systems have been identified. The detection of granulocyte specific antibodies may be made more difficult by the presence of HLA directed antibodies which occur in the same circumstances, after multiple transfusion and pregnancy, since similar methods are used in their detection.

The 'N' system of neutrophil specific antigens was first identified during the study of neonatal alloimmune neutropenia and is clinically the most important. So far five genetic loci controlling these antigens have been defined; A, B, C, D, E. The alleles are designated by numbers, for example, NA1 (Table 3.2). The method of detection most commonly used is leukoagglutination.

A second system of antigens, detected by granulocyte toxicity assay is called the human granulocyte associated system or HGA. This has 6 alleles, HGA-1, HGA-3a, 3b, 3c, 3d and 3e. A third system, Gr with two alleles Gr1 and Gr2, has also been detected. However, its restriction to granulocytes has been disputed. The clinical importance of HGA and Gr is less than that of the 'N' system.

The significance of granulocyte antigen-antibody reactions

Alloimmune reactions

NEONATAL ALLOIMMUNE NEUTROPENIA

This is analogous to haemolytic disease of the newborn. A mother carrying a fetus of different neutrophil type may have developed antibodies after antigenic exposure during previous childbirth or transfusion. If the antibodies are IgG, they can cross the placenta and destroy fetal granulocytes. The neonate may have severe neutropenia and develop bacterial infections. Antibiotics alone may be ineffective, and exchange transfusion to remove the antibody is required. Anti-NA1 and anti-NB1 are the most common antibodies found in this disorder.

ALLOIMMUNIZATION

Alloimmunization following transfusion of blood and blood products may occur. Severe febrile reactions occurring after repeated transfusion of blood, platelets or granulocytes may be due to granulocyte specific antibodies. Studies with indium-labelled granulocytes have demonstrated that infusion of incompatible granulocytes into patients with leukoagglutinins is followed by rapid sequestration by the liver, and failure of localization at infected body-sites. Leukoagglutinins may cause clumping of donor neutrophils in the pulmonary vasculature and pulmonary insufficiency. They may also activate the complement and the bradykinin systems causing tissue damage and vasodilation. The reactions are most severe during granulocyte transfusion where the antigenic load is highest.

During transfusion of blood febrile reactions due to granulocyte antibodies can be prevented by using white cell depleted blood. This is best done using the appropriate filters (page 57).

If granulocyte transfusion is required, HLA compatible blood is preferred; this avoids granulocyte destruction and reactions due to HLA antibodies. Granulocyte specific antibodies are excluded by 'crossmatching' the patient's serum against the donor's granulocytes using a leukoagglutination test. Often family members are used as donors.

Autoimmune reactions

(*a*) Neutropenia occurring during autoimmune disorders such as systemic lupus erythematosus, Felty's syndrome, thyroid disorders, immune thrombocytopenic purpura (ITP) and haemolytic anaemia can be caused by granulocyte specific autoantibodies. Angioimmunoblastic lymphadenopathy with dysproteinaemia can also be associated with immune neutropenia as well as a positive direct antiglobulin (Coombs') test.

(b)   Autoimmune neutropenia has also been reported in the absence of any other autoimmune problem. It can occur at any age, and in infancy may be confused with alloimmune neutropenia. Known neutrophil specific antibodies may be detected, but in some cases antibody is directed against as yet unidentified granulocyte antigens. It often follows viral infections and usually gets better spontaneously.

Drug-induced neutropenia

As in drug-induced haemolysis, drug-induced neutropenia may be due to the adsorption of drug/antibody immune complexes or the absorption of drug alone which then acts as a hapten inducing antibody production. True autoantibody production, possibly related to drug-related depression of suppressor T cell activity, also occurs. The drugs involved are aprindine and levamisole and their action is analogous to that of alpha-methyldopa in haemolytic anaemia. The part that the known neutrophil specific antigens play in drug-induced neutropenias is uncertain.

Platelet specific antigen systems

The important antigens displayed by platelets are shown in Table 3.3. Platelets carry adsorbed ABO but not rhesus antigens. Platelets carry HLA ABC (class I) antigens, but these are only weakly expressed and may be derived from the plasma. HLA class II antigens are not expressed and platelets are used to absorb class I antigen to prepare specific class II typing sera (Chapter 4).

Five platelet specific antigen systems are now known. Of these the Pl^A (or Zw) system is clinically the most important. There are two alleles, Pl^{A1} (or ZW(a)) found in 98% of individuals, and Pl^{A2} (or ZW(b)). The identification of these antigens is difficult because of the technical problems in isolating platelets without spontaneous aggregation, and in separating true platelet specific antibodies from HLA-directed antibodies as these often occur together after multiple platelet and blood product transfusions.

Table 3.3 Platelet specific antigens

Antigen	Frequency (%)
PI^{A1} (Zw^a)	98
PI^{A2} (Zw^b)	27
PI^{E1}	99.9
PI^{E2}	5
Ko^a	17
Ko^b	99
Bak^a	91
Duzo	22

(Modified from Schiffer, C A (1980) Clinical importance of antiplatelet antibody testing for the blood bank. In: *A Seminar on Antigens of Blood Cells.* American Association of Blood Banks, Washington D.C.)

Detection of platelet antibodies

Numerous assay systems for the detection of platelet antibody–antigen interactions have been devised. Platelet agglutination by platelet specific antibodies is unreliable because spontaneous aggregation is common. Indirect methods are therefore preferable. After exposure of platelets to antibody, they can be washed and treated with complement of anti-human globulin which will be fixed or 'consumed'; the amount consumed (indicated by reduced activity in a second indicator system containing antibody-coated red cells) is proportional to the amount of platelet-specific antibody. Alternatively anti-human globulin can be labelled using fluorescent compounds or radioisotopes which will allow detection of antibody coating the platelets. An enzyme-linked anti-human globulin can also be used to detect platelet antibodies by enzyme-linked immunoassay or Elisa. To detect non-HLA antibodies, platelets are pretreated with chloroquine which strips adsorbed HLA antigens.

The clinical significance of platelet antibodies

Alloimmune platelet destruction

NEONATAL PURPURA

Neonatal purpura may occur if a mother carrying a fetus of different platelet antigen type develops the corresponding IgG antibody. If sufficient antibodies cross the placenta, the infant suffers from thrombocytopenia. This is usually mild, resolving as the maternal antibody is catabolized. In severe cases compatible platelets need to be transfused. In most cases the neonatal platelet antigen involved is Pl^{A1} and, since 98% of the general population are Pl^{A1} positive, the most readily available donor is the mother (who must be Pl^{A1} negative). In some cases only HLA antibodies have been detected in the mother.

POST-TRANSFUSION PURPURA

Post-transfusion purpura develops 5–10 days after blood transfusion and is due to development of antibodies to the antigens on contaminating platelets. The recipient's own platelets are probably destroyed by aggregation with the antibody-coated donor platelets. The antigen system involved is usually Pl^{A1}, the recipient being Pl^{A1} negative. The thrombocytopenia usually resolves in 2–4 weeks but may be severe, requiring treatment by plasmapheresis.

PLATELET ANTIBODIES FOLLOWING TRANSFUSION

The transfusion of blood or blood products containing platelets may cause immunization against platelet specific antigens not present in the donor (see above). Transfusions may also immunize the recipient against HLA antigens, because white cells express HLA antigens strongly—they are more potent HLA immunogens than platelets. However, HLA-directed antibodies are frequently the cause of febrile reactions and poor platelet increments following platelet transfusions. If the corrected platelet increment (CPI) is less than 10×10^9 one hour after transfusion of 6 units to an adult, immunization is probable and HLA compatible family donors should be sought.

$$CIP = \frac{(\text{Post-transfusion count} - \text{pretransfusion count}) \times \text{surface area (m}^2)}{\text{Number of platelets transfused}}$$

Immunization to HLA antibodies can be confirmed by the detection of lymphocytotoxins in the recipient's serum (see page 41). The presence of platelet-specific antibodies is detected by one of the methods outlined above, using donor platelets and a panel of platelets of known specificity.

Autoimmune platelet destruction

Autoimmune thrombocytopenic purpura probably accounts for most cases of spontaneous thrombocytopenia previously called 'idiopathic'.

The antibody is usually IgG and is not directed against any of the known platelet antigens. There is an elevated level of platelet-associated IgG in the majority of cases, but free IgG platelet antibody is not always detectable in the serum. Since the antigen involved is not known but appears to be present on most platelets, platelet transfusion is not possible. This is analogous to autoimmune haemolysis. Treatment is by immunosuppression with steroids; splenectomy may be useful in some patients.

SYSTEMIC LUPUS ERYTHEMATOSUS

Thrombocytopenia developing in association with systemic lupus erythematosus is sometimes due to platelet directed antibodies, but it has recently been recognized that the 'lupus anticoagulant' may also be responsible. This is an antibody directed against phospholipid that is responsible for the 'false positive' results in the VDRL test for syphilis in these patients. The interaction between the antibody and platelet phospholipid is thought to induce platelet activation and aggregation. Thus despite thrombocytopenia there is increased tendency to thrombosis.

Autoimmune thrombocytopenia may also occur with autoimmune haemolytic anaemia (Evan's syndrome) as well as with the lymphoproliferative disorders. In the latter the appearance of such antibodies can precede the disease by some years.

Further reading

McCullough, J (1980) Granulocyte antigen systems and antibodies and their clinical significance, *Human Pathology*, **14**, 228.

Lalezari, P. (1977) Neutrophil specific antigens: immunology and clinical significance. In: *The Granulocyte: Function and Clinical Utilization, Progress in Clinical and Biological Research*. Eds. Greenwalt, T J, Jamieson, G A. A R Liss, New York, p 209.

Verheut, F W A, von dem Borne, A E G K and von Noord-Bokhorst, J C (1978) Serological immunochemical and immunocytological properties of granulocyte antibodies. *Vox Sang*, **35**, 294.

McCullough, J, Clay, M E, Priest, J R (1981) A comparison of methods for detecting leukocyte antibodies in autoimmune neutropenia. *Transfusion*, **21**, 483.

Lalezari, P, Radel, E (1974) Neutrophil specific antigens: immunology and clinical significance. *Seminars in Haematology*, **11**, 281.

Miller, W, Harmon J (1983) Platelet serology and transfusion. *Human Pathology*, 14, 221.

Karpatkin, S (1980) Autoimmune thrombocytopenic purpura. *Blood*, 56, 329.

Le Roux, G, Pourrait, J L, Lepandry, C, Aufeuvre, J P, Le Floch, A, Baudelot, J, Lorthaolary, P (1981) Le purpura post-transfusionnel. *Rev. Franc Transfus Immunohemat*, 24, 211.

4 The HLA system and the major histocompatibility complex

The HLA system or 'Human Leucocyte Associated' system of antigens is a group of highly polymorphic antigens found on the surface of most nucleated human cells. Because these antigens were first recognized on white cells they were named leucocyte associated. Their importance lies in the fact that HLA-antigenic differences between individuals is responsible for graft rejection when tissue is transplanted from one person to another. They may also be associated with host defence against malignancy and some infections.

Genetic control of the HLA system

The HLA system of antigens is controlled by a group of closely linked genetic loci called the major histocompatibility complex, present on the short arm of chromosome 6. There are four loci of major importance named HLA A, B, C and D. The antigens of the HLA ABC loci are known as class I, while the HLA D antigens are class II. The complement components coded for on chromosome 6 between the class I and class II loci are called class III. It has recently been recognized that there are at least three loci within HLA-D: DR, DQ(DC) and DP(SB) (Fig. 4.1). They are highly polymorphic and there is a large

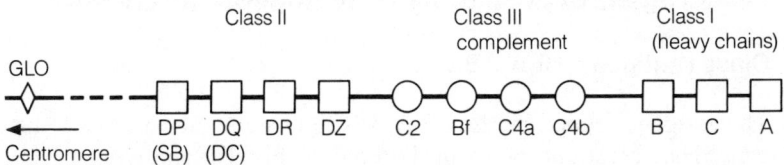

Fig. 4.1 A schematic representation of the loci of the histocompatibility complex on chromosome 6.

number of possible alternatives or alleles of HLA A, B, C and D which an individual may possess. For example, there are over 40 possible alleles at the B locus, and new alleles are still being discovered (see Table 4.1).

An individual inherits one set of alleles (A, B, C, D) on the paternal chromosome and a second set on the maternal chromosome. As the four loci are closely linked the four alleles segregate together and the whole 'haplotype' is inherited intact. However, if, during meiosis to form the gametes, crossing over between the homologous chromosomes occurs, exchange of genetic material may take place. The closer two genetic loci are on the chromosome, the less likely it is that they will be separated during this process of crossing over or 'genetic recombination'. Examination of the frequencies of individual HLA genes and the frequencies of certain haplotypes shows that some gene combinations are much more common than expected. For example, the alleles HLA A1 and B8 are found together five times more frequently in Caucasian populations than would be expected if they had been randomly associated over many generations. Such genes are said to be in 'linkage disequilibrium'.

Crossing over occurs relatively infrequently, so for example, if an individual with the haplotypes w/x (w representing the HLA genes on one chromosome and x those on the other) mates with an individual with the haplotypes y/z, four possible combinations can occur in their offspring: w/y, w/z, x/y, x/z. There is consequently only a one-in-four chance that any two offspring will be identical (Fig. 4.2).

The fact that linkage disequilibrium exists between certain genetic loci can be useful if for technical reasons the assignment of an individual's D type is difficult. Fortunately certain genes of the D locus are in linkage disequilibrium with the loci determining the structure of certain complement components. Therefore by analysing the individual's 'complotype' the D type may often be deduced.

The antigens of the major histocompatibility complex

Class I antigens: HLA-ABC

The antigens defined by the HLA-ABC loci are known as class I antigens. They are found on all nucleated cells, platelets and reticulocytes. They are not present on spermatozoa or placental trophoblast. Some HLA antigens may be weakly expressed on red cells, for example HLA-

Table 4.1 HLA specificities

Class I				Class II			
A	**B** (with Bw4)	**B** (with Bw6)	**C**	**D**	**DR**	**DQ**	**DP**
A1	B5 {Bw51, Bw52}	B7	Cw1	Dw1	DR1	DQw1	DPw1
A2	B13	B8	Cw2	Dw2	DR2	DQw2	DPw2
A3	B17 {Bw57, Bw58}	B14 {Bw64, Bw65}	Cw3	Dw3	*DR3	DQw3	DPw3
A9 {A23, A24}	B27	B18	Cw4	Dw4	†DR4		DPw4
A10 {A25, A26}	B37	B22 {Bw54, Bw55, Bw56}	Cw5	Dw5			DPw5
A11	B47	B35	Cw6	Dw6 {Dw18, Dw19}	*DR5 {DRw11, DRw12}		DPw6
Aw19 {A29, A30, A31, A32, Aw33}	Bw53	B40 {Bw60, Bw61}	Cw7	Dw7 {Dw11, Dw17}	*DRw6 {DRw13, DRw14}		
A28	Bw59	Bw41	Cw8	Dw8	†DR7		
Aw34		Bw42		Dw9	*DRw8		
Aw36		Bw46		Dw10	†DRw9		
Aw43		Bw48		Dw12	DRw10		
		Bw67		Dw13			
		Bw70 {Bw71, Bw72}		Dw14			
		Bw73		Dw15			
				Dw16			

Co-expression box (B subtypes determined by Bw4/Bw6):

with Bw4		with Bw6
B44	← B12 →	B45
Bw63	← B15 →	Bw62
B38	← B16 →	B39
B49	← B21 →	Bw50

DR footnotes:
* with DRW52
† with Drw53

Subtypes of certain HLA specificities are indicated following the brackets. All B-specificities occur with either Bw4 or Bw6 as shown. With B12, B15, B16 and B21 the subtype is determined by the co-expression of Bw4 or Bw6. For example when B12 occurs with Bw4 the subtype is B44, while B12 with Bw6 is B45. Similarly certain DR specificities occur with either DRw52 or DRw53 as indicated.

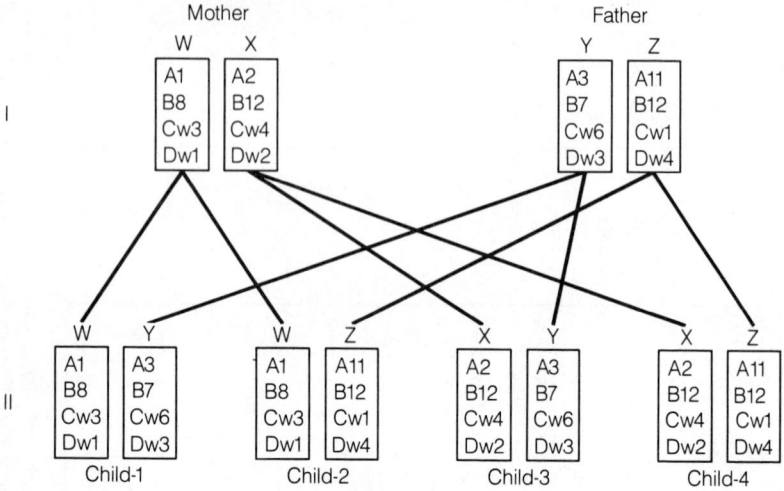

Fig. 4.2 The inheritance of the HLA haplotypes giving a 1:4 chance of siblings being identical.

B7 (Bga), B17 (Bgb) and A28 (Bgc). During some lymphoproliferative and leukaemic disorders, and very rarely in some normal individuals, the antigens are strongly expressed on the red cells. For this reason blood group typing sera should be free of HLA antibodies. It is very fortunate that in general HLA antigens are not significantly expressed on the red cells, otherwise blood transfusion would be severely limited.

The structure of the HLA molecules

Class I antigens are composed of two non-covalently linked polypeptides, one heavy and one light chain (Fig. 4.3A). The heavy chains are the product of the HLA A, B and C genes and these are structurally polymorphic. They have a molecular weight of 44,000, are glycosylated and are attached through the plasma membrane by a hydrophobic portion. The antigenic sites defining HLA A, B and C types reside in these polypeptide chains, each different antigenic type being represented on a separate HLA molecule in the cell membrane. In general C-locus antigens are relatively weakly expressed.

The light chain is β_2 microglobulin and has a molecular weight of 12,000. Unlike HLA A, B, C and D determinants, it is a product

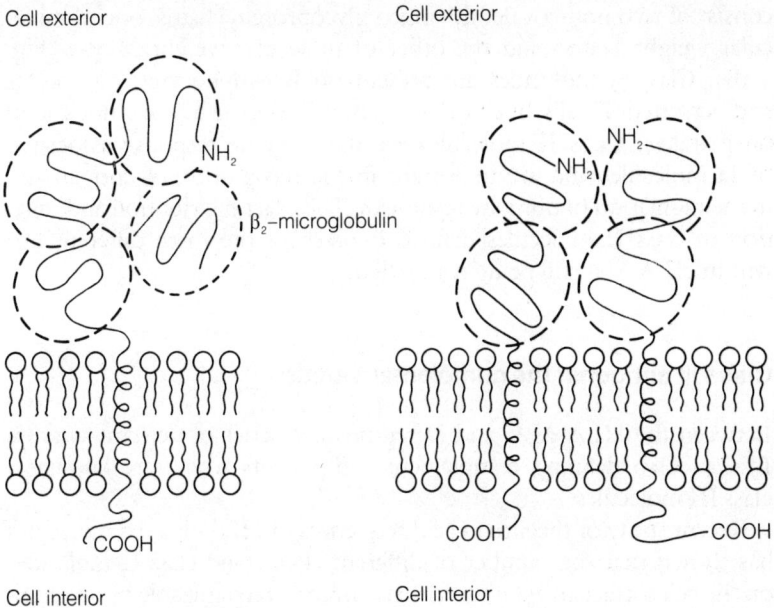

Fig. 4.3   Diagrammatic representation of the HLA antigens. Like other trans-membrane proteins there are internal and external hydrophylic regions, joined by a helical transmembrane hydrophobic section. This anchors the protein to the membrane. Each of the HLA antigens probably consists of four external domains. (A) Class I antigens, HLA ABC, consist of one heavy chain, which anchors the protein to the cell membrane to which is joined the light chain, β_2-microglobulin. (B) Class II antigens consist of two chains, α and β, each anchored to the membrane and each carrying their own antigenic determinants.

of a gene on chromosome 15. Cells that lack β_2 microglobulin such as the 'Daudi' cell-line, cannot express the HLA-ABC genes. β_2 microglobulin is found free in the serum and its level increases in some lympho-proliferative disorders.

The class I antigens are those recognized by cytotoxic effector T lymphocytes during graft rejection and the elimination of virus infected cells.

Class II antigens: the HLA-D locus

The HLA-D locus consists of several closely linked loci: DP(SB), DQ(DC), DR, and DZ. These genes define class II molecules which consist of two non-covalently linked glycoprotein chains, one of molecular weight 33,000 and the other of molecular weight 28,000 (Fig. 4.3B). Class II molecules are present on B lymphocytes, monocytes and activated T cells but not on resting T cells. They are not found on platelets. Class II molecules are the immune response associated or Ia molecules and are important in the recognition of antigen and in the regulation of immune responses. The exact distribution and function of class II molecules defined by each of the three different loci within HLA-D is still being researched.

Class III antigens: the complement locus

Between the HLA-ABC and D regions is a series of determinants C2 Bf C4a C4b defining complement components which are known as class III molecules.

Recent study of the amino acid sequences of HLA-defined molecules has shown that the number of different class I and class II molecules on the cell surface may be twice that currently recognizable by serological and cellular typing techniques (page 41). It has also been discovered that for both class I and class II molecules, those parts near to the cell membrane show striking amino acid sequence homology to the immunoglobulin constant region. This may be of functional significance since HLA-defined molecules have been shown to bind antigens, viruses and drugs. The phenonemon may be involved in antigen recognition and immune regulation.

The marked genetic polymorphism within the HLA system may be related to the role of these molecules in antigen (e.g. virus) presentation and recognition. It is of advantage to a species if there is a vast array of molecules that can perform this function, since there is more chance of some individuals surviving an epidemic. The phenomenon of tissue transplant rejection and graft versus host disease may be explained by the theory that allogeneic HLA molecules are perceived as 'altered self' (that is self-HLA plus antigen).

The laboratory assignment of HLA types

Technical details are beyond the scope of this book and the reader is referred to further reading at the end of the chapter.

HLA-ABC typing

The class I antigens were first discovered when sera from multiparous women were found to contain antibodies to some allogeneic lymphocytes. Today panels of sera from multiparous women, or patients who have had organ transplants, which are of known HLA-ABC specificity are available for tissue typing. The sera are incubated with the test lymphocytes in the presence of complement and a dye (either trypan blue or eosin). If this results in the killing of a significant number of the test lymphocytes (indicated by uptake of the dye), then they bear the antigen for which the serum was specific. This is called the microlymphocytotoxicity test and is an example of serological typing.

D-locus typing

The antigens defined by the HLA-D loci are known as lymphocyte-activating determinants, each locus probably controls antigens that function differently during the immune response, and there may well be other, as yet undiscovered, lymphocyte-activating determinants within and possibly also outside the MHC.

Early in the development of tissue typing it was recognized that, if unseparated lymphocyte populations from two different individuals were mixed together, they were mutually stimulated to become actively dividing 'blast' cells. It was later recognized that during this 'mixed lymphocyte culture' (MLC), B lymphocyte antigens (determined by the D locus) elicit a response from certain T lymphocyte subpopulations of the other individual. The degree of response can be measured by the incorporation of ^{3}H-thymidine. The mixed lymphocyte culture test has the disadvantage of being lengthy, and indicating only that there is a difference in D type, not its specificity.

One way of adapting this principle for cell typing is to use panels of B cells from individuals born of consanguinous marriages. These 'homozygous' typing cells (HTC) of known specificity are inactivated with mitomycin C, and incubated with test T-lymphocytes in the presence of tritiated thymidine. If stimulation occurs, the test T cells will become active and take up radioactive thymidine during DNA synthesis. If no reaction occurs (provided known positive controls are included), it can be assumed that the test cells are of the same type as the HTC used. A panel of HTC is used and therefore both loci can be assigned. This is an example of 'negative' typing.

A second adaptation of the MLC for D typing is the primed lymphocyte test (PLT). T cells homozygous at the D locus are prestimulated with inactivated known B cells, of a specific different D type. They are then kept in culture for 14 days. When restimulated with inactivated test B lymphocytes, a rapid 'secondary' proliferative response will only occur in the T cells if the test B cells are of the same HLA-D type as the priming B cells. This is an example of a 'positive' typing reaction.

Serological typing for HLA-D loci

Sera from multiparous women can be adsorbed using platelets which express only class I antigens. The sera can then be used to detect D locus (class II) specificity. It is uncertain whether HTC typing and serological typing methods recognize exactly the same antigenic structure on the D antigen, the antigen defined by HTC is therefore called, for example, HLA-D1 and its serological counterpart HLA-DR1, DR signifying D-'related'. However, recent serological and biochemical studies have defined the relationships between the different D antigens.

Clinical significance of the HLA antigens

Transplantation of solid organs

Cells of the kidney, heart or liver carry class I antigens (HLA-ABC) antigens, which act as the targets of cytotoxic cells and antibodies when transplanted into a non-HLA identical recipient. Even when cadaver or live sibling donor tissue is HLA-ABC identical with the recipient rejection may still occur, presumably due to other as yet undefined antigens. Thus in all cases the recipient requires immunosuppression; only when a truly identical organ is available from a monozygotic twin is this unnecessary.

Having secured a donor as closely HLA matched as possible, the presence of HLA specific antibodies of the recipient's serum is excluded by cross-matching it against donor lymphocytes in a lymphocytotoxicity test. The presence of such antibodies is more likely in a patient who has had numerous blood transfusions, as contaminating white cells carry HLA antigen, and will result in hyperacute rejection. A positive cross-match therefore means that the organ is unsuitable.

Another test that predicts graft survival is the MLC, which defines differences at the D locus. If the donor and recipient lymphocytes react strongly in the MLC and are not D/DR identical, graft survival may be less good. For cadaver donors only DR typing is possible in the time available. The D locus determines immune responsiveness but the exact reason why it is of importance in solid organ transplants is not known. It is probable that D-locus compatibility is more important than HLA-ABC identity.

The transfusion of less than about 10 units of blood prior to organ transplant has been found to confer an increased survival of a subsequent HLA matched graft, when compared with recipients who have not been transfused. A number of theories have been put forward to explain this phenomenon. Transfusion may expose them to a range of HLA antigens, eliciting antibody responses. When the serum is then cross-matched against the donor lymphocytes, organs with the HLA type to which the patient has already made a response are identified, and those to which the patient is relatively unresponsive are selected. Thus transfusion in small amounts may act as a screening process for antigens to which the recipient is able to make vigorous responses. Alternatively tolerance to certain antigens may be induced during transfusion.

A further hypothesis is that transfusion acts as a primary antigenic stimulus and the transplanted organ then elicits a vigorous secondary response just at the time when maximum immunosuppressive treatment is operating. This effectively deletes the immunoreactive clones. If proved, this theory would imply that timing is crucial to the outcome of the transplant, and that immunization to HLA antigens and subsequent immune suppression could be deliberately planned as an event before transplantation with obvious benefit to the patient.

Bone marrow transplantation

During selection for bone marrow transplantation (BMT) the previously discussed considerations apply. Prior to BMT the patient is conditioned with cyclophosphamide and TBI or other regimen. These produce severe immune suppression in the recipient and graft rejection is less of a problem in BMT. Bone marrow graft rejection occurs in patients who have less intensive conditioning regimens. However, marrow is itself immunocompetent, the donor T cells being able to mount a graft versus host response against recipient HLA antigens. Therefore only HLA-AB(C) identical donors whose lymphocytes react negatively with those of the recipient in the MLC are used. However, it has recently become possible to prevent and treat graft versus host reactions and complete HLA (four locus) identity is not always required (p. 171).

Transfusion prior to bone marrow transplant is often unavoidable in patients with leukaemia. Fortunately they receive immunosuppressive therapy and transfusion is less likely to sensitize these patients against HLA antigens. For patients with aplastic anaemia who are potential bone marrow recipients transfusion should be avoided.

It is believed that class II (D-locus defined) differences between donor and recipient are the most important in predicting the outcome of marrow transplantation. The class II antigens stimulate allogeneic helper T lymphocytes which then induce cellular and humoral responses, to both class II and class I molecules, by cytotoxic T lymphocytes and B lymphocytes. Because of this, attempts are often made to reduce the chance of sensitization to class II antigens in the pretransplantation period by depleting all red cells and platelets of granulocytes and lymphocytes prior to transfusion. This is best achieved by centrifugation and filtration (page 55). Frozen reconstituted red cells were previously advocated but may be contaminated with leucocyte fragments and are less suitable.

These manipulations are particularly important for those patients with aplastic anaemia in whom transfusion is unavoidable. In all cases the transfusion of blood products from the potential donor is contraindicated, since this may result in sensitization to HLA and non-HLA antigen differences, which cannot be recognized by currently available techniques but result in graft rejection or graft versus host disease.

Platelet and granulocyte transfusion

Febrile reactions and failure of therapeutic response to these components is frequently due to HLA antibodies (page 136).

Diseases associated with HLA type

It has been found that individuals of certain HLA types suffer from certain diseases more frequently than the general population. These disorders are often of multifactorial causation, and associated with defective immune regulation. The MHC antigens may play a role in facilitating invasion of a pathogen, or they may be antigenically similar to a pathogen, and unable to make it the target of an effective immune response. In many cases the D locus may determine an aberration in immune response or regulation. A table of diseases associated with HLA antigens is given (Table 4.2).

Table 4.2   HLA types and disease associations

Disease	Antigen
Ankylosing spondylitis	B27
Reiter's syndrome	B27
Post-infective arthritis	B27
Acute anterior uveitis	B27
Behçet's disease	B5
Congenital adrenal hyperplasia	B47
Dermatitis herpetiformis	DR3
SLE	DR3
Pemphigus	DR4
Goodpasture's syndrome	DR2
Myasthenia gravis	DR3
Sicca syndrome	DR3
Coeliac disease	DR3
Subacute thyroiditis	B35
Rheumatoid arthritis	DR4
gold nephropathy	DR3
(most common haplocyte: B8, Cw7, DR3)	
post D-penicillamine	
myasthenia gravis	DR1; DR7
Addison's disease	DR3
Haemochromatosis	A3; B14
Multiple sclerosis	DR2
Chronic active hepatitis	DR3
Type 1 diabetes	DR4; DR3
Hyperthyroidism	DR3
Psoriasis	Cw6
Hodgkin's disease	HLA-linked

Further reading

Bodmer, W F, (Ed.) (1978) The HLA system. *British Medical Bulletin*, volume 34, no. 3 (whole volume).

Bodmer, J, Bodmer, W (1984) Histocompatibility 1984. *Immunology Today*, **5**, 251–254.

Bender, K (1984) The HLA system. *Biotest Bulletin*, **2**, 63–116.

Svejgaard, A, Platz P, Ryder, L P (1983) HLA and disease 1982—a survey. *Immunological Reviews*, **70**, 193–218.

Terasaki, P (1984) The beneficial transfusion effect on kidney graft survival attributed to clonal detection. *Transplantation*, **37**, 119–125.

Yunis, E J, Awdeh, Z, Raum, D, Alperc, A (1984) The MHC in human bone marrow transplantation. *Clinics in Haematology*, **12**, 641–680.

5 Red cell transfusion

Transfusion involves the collection, storage, processing and administration of blood and its various products.

Blood is collected into plastic blood collection bags containing an anticoagulant. Nowadays most of the blood taken is processed as outlined in Figure 5.1 and it is important that the right collection pack is used to enable fractionation to be carried out in a closed system avoiding the introduction of infection. An example of a modern taking set is shown in Figure 5.2

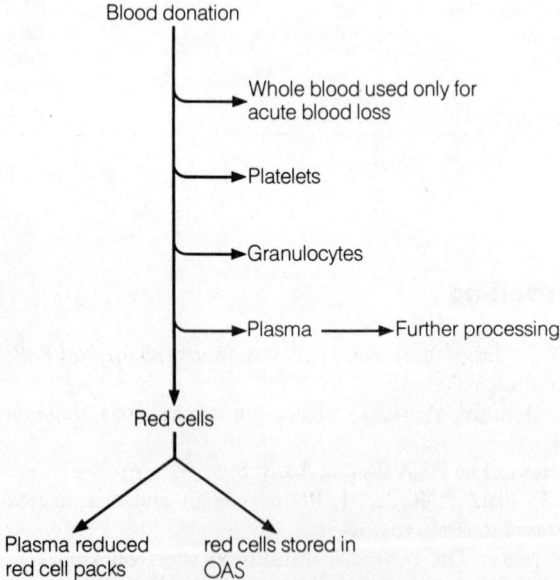

Blood donation

Whole blood used only for acute blood loss

Platelets

Granulocytes

Plasma ——→ Further processing

Red cells

Plasma reduced red cell packs

red cells stored in OAS

Fig. 5.1 Outline of various fractions of blood available for transfusion.

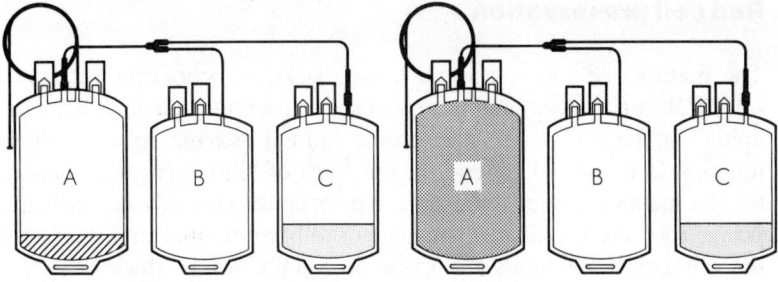

1. Triple OPTIMAL ADDITIVE Blood Collection System as supplied. Unit A contains 63ml CPD anticoagulant. Unit C contains 100ml SAG-M. solution.

2. Collect 450ml blood in unit A.

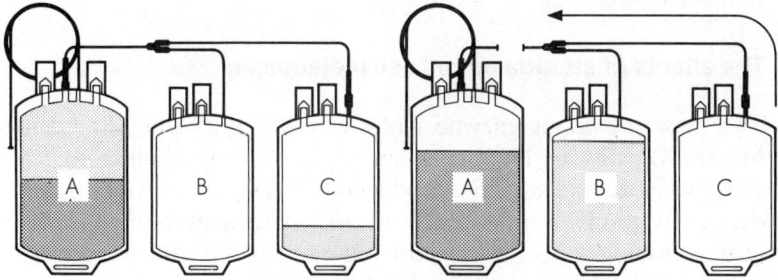

3. Centrifuge to separate out red cells.

4. Express plasma into unit B. Transfer SAG-M solution from C to A. Seal and disconnect unit A, which now contains red cell mass suspended in SAG-M.

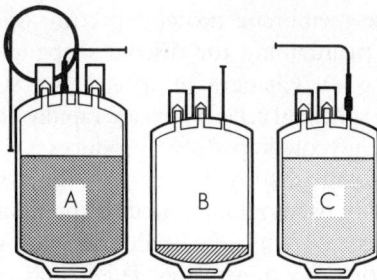

5. Centrifuge unit B. Express platelet-poor plasma into unit C, leaving platelet concentrate suspended in 50ml of plasma in B. Seal both units and disconnect.

NOTE. Cryoprecipitate may be prepared as an alternative to platelets.

Fig. 5.2 Triple blood collection system. (*Courtesy of Fenwal/Travenol*)

Red cell preservation

The mature red cell is non-nucleated, lacks mitochondria and ribosomes. It is therefore unable to synthesize proteins, adenine, haem or lipids. In the red cell there are only limited enzyme systems whose function is to provide energy in the form of high energy phosphates for the maintenance of the ionic integrity of the cell, provide reducing power to prevent oxidant damage to the haemoglobin molecules and red cell membrane lipids and maintain 2,3DPG levels which modulate oxygen delivery. During the 120-day life span of the cell the activity of many of these enzymes declines. In the non-physiological milieu of the various storage media, and at 4°C their activity declines even more quickly. Therefore it is not surprising that the viability and function of red cells is impaired by storage.

The effects of storage on red cell metabolism

The most important enzyme pathway is the glycolytic (Embden—Meyerhof) pathway (Fig. 5.3), whereby glucose is metabolized to pyruvate and lactic acid with the production of ATP and NADH. Energy derived from ATP is necessary for the maintenance of the high intracellular concentration of potassium (90–100 mmol/l) and low concentration of sodium (5–15 mmol/l) against the steep concentration gradients with plasma. The ATP levels fall on storage and, as it reaches 5–15% of its initial value, sodium enters the cell and the osmotic fragility increases. This reduces red cell viability on subsequent transfusion. High energy phosphate compounds are also responsible for the phosphorylation of the membrane protein spectrin. Spectrin is the main 'skeletal' protein, maintaining the discoid shape and deformibility of the red cell (page 4). Changes in spectrin on storage lead to the formation of rigid spherical cells, which are rapidly destroyed *in vivo*.

A bypass of the glycolytic pathway produces 2,3DPG: 2,3DPG falls more rapidly on storage than ATP (Fig. 5.4). It plays a role in reducing the oxygen affinity of haemoglobin, modulating tissue oxygen delivery. Full oxygen delivery capacity of 2,3DPG depleted stored blood takes 4–12 hours to restore after transfusion. This is only of great importance in massive or exchange transfusion. It may explain why the beneficial effects of such transfusions appear to be delayed. These changes have been minimized by improvements in the anticoagulant/preservative solution used. All the anticoagulants (Table 5.1) are based on citrate which chelates calcium, and also provide an energy substrate for the

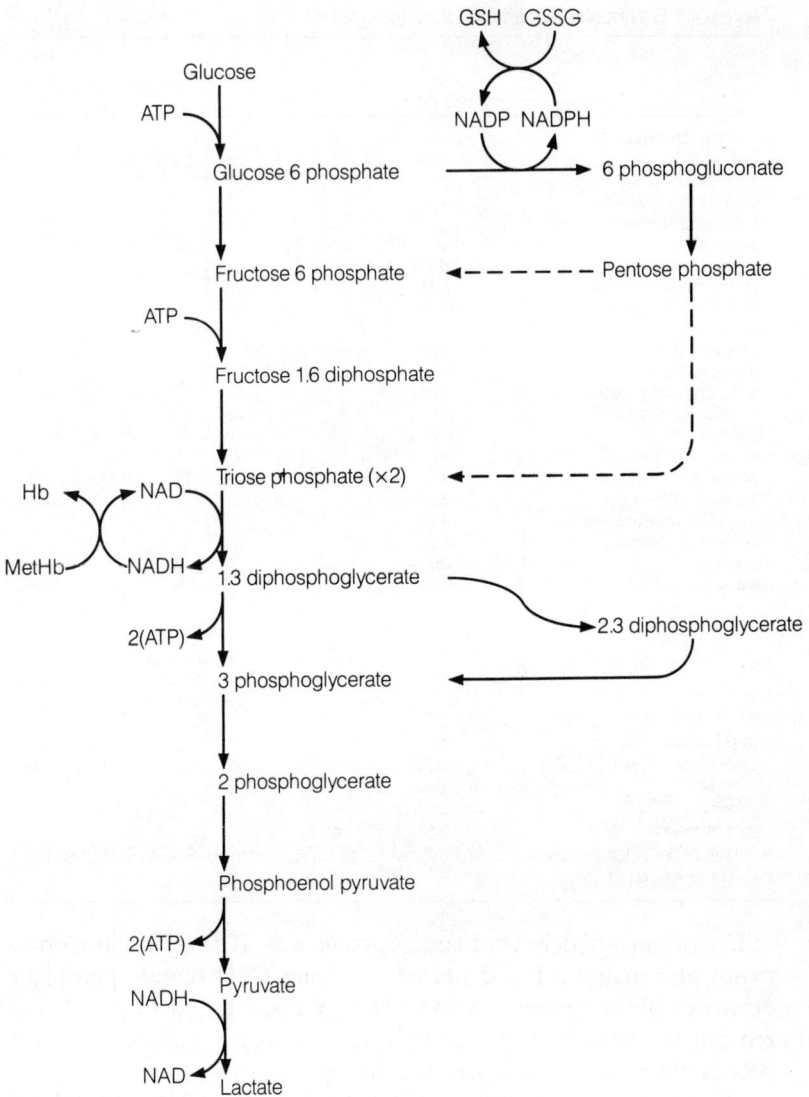

Fig. 5.3   The glycolytic (Embden-Meyerhof) pathway.

glycolytic pathway as some form of glucose. The minimum standard that any anticoagulant solution must meet is that after the stated maximum period of storage the red cell survival 24 hours post transfusion must be over 70%.

Table 5.1   Composition of anticoagulant solutions

	g/l	ph	ml/100ml blood	Storage 4 –6°C (days)
Acid Citrate Dextrose ACD				
citric acid	8.0	5	15	21
trisodium citrate H_2O	22.0			
dextrose monohydrate	24.5			
Citrate phosphate dextrose CPD				
citric acid	3.27	5.6	14	21
trisodium citrate H_2O	26.3			
sodium dihydrogen phosphate	2.22			
dextrose monohydrate	25.5			
CPD A1 (CPD A)				
citric acid	3.27	5.6	14	35
trisodium citrate H_2O	26.3			
sodium dihydrogen phosphate	2.22			
dextrose monohydrate	31.9			
adenine	0.2752			
CPD A2				
citric acid	3.27	5.6	14	35
trisodium citrate H_2O	26.3			
sodium dihydrogen phosphate	2.22			
dextrose monohydrate	44.6			
adenine	0.5504			
Heparin	75,000 iu/l saline		6	48 hours

Red cell additive solutions			amount added to one unit packed cells (ml)	
SAG-M (Fenwall)				
dextrose monohydrate	9.0	6.0	100	35
adenine	0.169			
mannitol	5.25			
sodium chloride	8.77 (150 mEq)			

Various other additive solutions are available: ADSOL (Fenwal), PAGGS (Biotest), Formula 052 (B) (Tuta).

The original widely used anticoagulant was ACD (acid citrate dextrose) pH5 giving a blood pH of 7.0. Later CPD (citrate phosphate dextrose) pH5.6 giving a blood pH of 7.2 was found to give better red cell viability. Red cell 2,3DPG was also better maintained. CPD became the preferred anticoagulant during the 1970s.

The addition of adenine to CPD was known to improve red cell viability by providing the nucleotide for ATP synthesis during storage. However, its use was delayed by fears of renal toxicity, since it has an insoluble metabolite. However, at the levels used no adverse effects have been demonstrated. Adenine-containing preservatives have been in widespread use since around 1980. CPD-A1 contains 0.25 mmol adenine/l, and CPD-A2 0.5 mmol/l. The addition of adenine allows

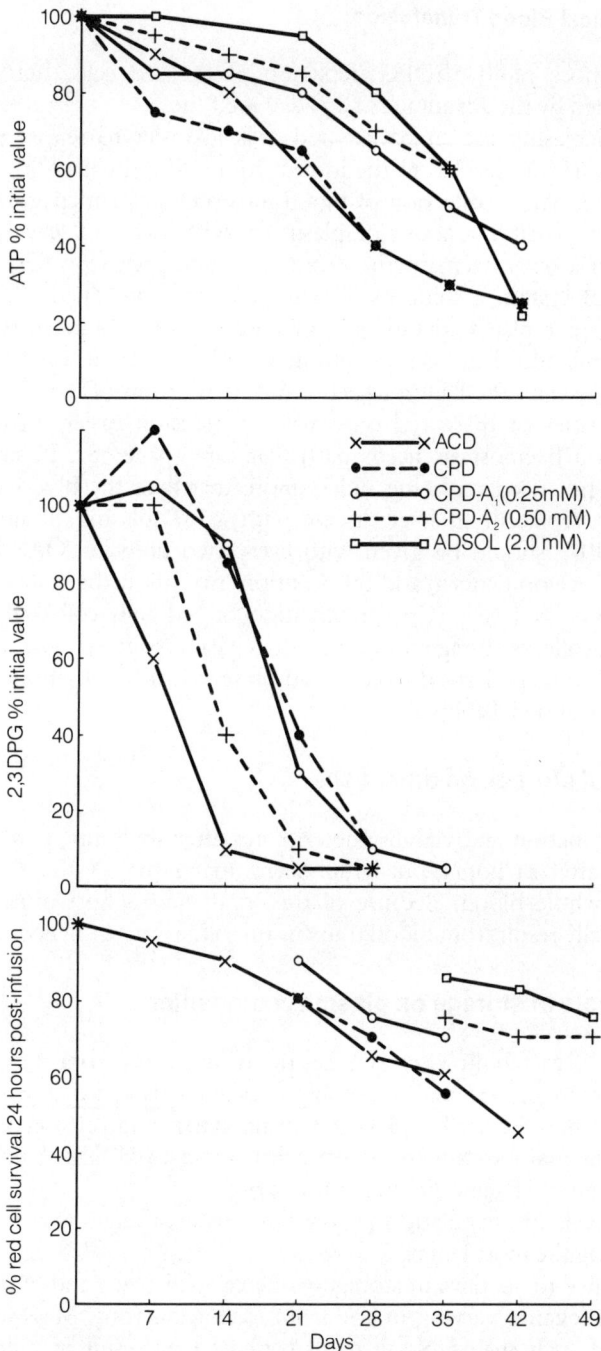

Fig. 5.4 Changes in ATP, 2, 3 DPG and 24 hour red cell survival.

slightly more rapid 2,3DPG depletion of the red cells, but this is outweighed by the advantage of a 35-day shelf-life.

The increasing use of packed red cells in order to release plasma for fractionation, has led to the introduction of 'optimal additive solutions' OAS. After collection of blood into standard anticoagulant the maximum possible amount of plasma is withdrawn to leave packed cells with a 90% haematocrit. From a satellite pack (Fig. 5.2) within the closed system a solution of saline adenine and glucose 'SAG' is added. This replaces adenine and glucose and reduces haematocrit to 60%. Some additives also contain mannitol, e.g. ADSOL or SAG-M (Table 5.1). The shelf life of such red cells is 35 days. The good flow characteristics of these red cells make transfusion easier. In massive transfusion haemostasis needs particular care (page 70). Plasma proteins do not need replacing unless more than half the blood volume has been replaced. In liver disease with a low plasma albumin one unit of PPF should be given with every two units of 'OAS blood'. Further developments in additive solutions may allow the 'rejuvenation' of outdated red cells. Cryopreservation of red cells collected in the usual way allows storage for at least three years (page 53). The different red cell products derived from liquid preserved red cells are described on page 53 and in Table 5.2.

Effects of storage on other cells

Platelet function and viability deteriorates after six hours, granulocyte viability after 24 hours, but lymphocytes may remain viable for many days in whole blood. Because of this, graft versus host disease may occasionally result from blood transfusion to the fetus or ill neonate.

The effects of storage on plasma composition

Because of metabolic compromise, potassium leaks from the red cell during storage, and may reach high levels. This is because red cell K^+ is 20 times the level in plasma. During massive transfusion of stored blood this may be dangerous (page 70). Plasma pH falls slightly during storage and haemoglobin in plasma rises.

The levels of coagulation factors fall during storage, factors V and VIII being the most labile.

After five to six days in storage white cells, platelets and fibrin form microaggregates, varying in size from 10–200 microns. Massive transfusion of such stored blood to ill patients may result in pulmonary

Table 5.2   Red cell products

Product	Volume (ml)	Haematocrit (%)	Shelf life (days)	Indication
Whole blood				
CPD	500	39	21	Massive bleeding
CPD-A	500	39	35	Massive bleeding
Heparin	450	45	2	Neonatal exchange, cardiopulmonary bypass
Plasma reduced				
Blood	340	60	21–35*	General transfusion
Red cells in optimal additive solutions				
SAG-M or ADSOL)	340	60	35	General transfusion with good flow characteristics
Packed				
red cells	300	70	21–35*	Chronic anaemia
Washed				
red cells	300	70	12 hours	Patients with PNH or with anti-IgA
Frozen				
red cells†	300	70	12 hours	Patients with rare blood groups or white cell antibodies
Leucocyte-poor red cells see Table 5.3				

* Depends on anticoagulant used
† Available only in some centres

insufficiency, renal or cerebral impairment. In-line microaggregate filters with a pore size of 20–40 μm are designed to prevent this, but are unsuitable for use during platelet transfusion.

Plasticizers may leach out of storage packs into lipids. They may accumulate in the recipient. Experience over the years suggests that no immediate harm results but the long-term effects are not known.

Cryopreservation of red cells

During the freezing of mammalian cells, ice crystals form. If the freezing rate is rapid, they form intracellularly, increasing the concentration of the remaining cell contents with resultant influx of water and cell damage. At slow rates of freezing ice cyrstals form extracellularly, effectively concentrating the remaining extracellular fluid, resulting in increased osmotic pressure and intracellular dehydration, which also reduces cell viability. Therefore in order to freeze cells without reducing subsequent viability the rate of cooling must be carefully controlled and a cryoprotectant which minimizes the crystal formation must be used.

Standard packed red cells, collected in polyolefin plastic packs which resist low temperatures, are mixed with the cryopreservative glycerol. For rapid freezing rates this is used at 3.8M concentration and the cells are stored in liquid nitrogen; for slower freezing rates a higher concentation, 6.2M, is used, and storage is in mechanical freezers at −80°C. Frozen red cells can be stored for many years.

When required the frozen red cells are rapidly thawed at 40°C and washed in hypertonic saline to remove glycerol. Repeated washing in successively more dilute saline is performed, the cells being suspended in isotonic saline or balanced salt solution for transfusion. The process of reconstitution takes around one hour and involves breaching the pack, risking contamination. The red cells slowly lyse after reconstitution. For both these reasons the blood must be used within 12 hours.

In general the properties of reconstituted cryopreserved red cells depend on their state at the time of freezing. Therefore they should be frozen within five days of collection. Up to 50% of their ATP can be lost during prefreeze storage and a further 5–25% is lost during processing; 2,3DPG is even less well preserved. Recently it has been suggested that outdated liquid-stored red cells may be rejuvenated by manoeuvres to replenish ATP and 2,3DPG and subsequently cryopreserved. The 24 hour survival of cryopreserved red cells after transfusion is 90%. Less than 5% of the white cells of the original donation are present, but the remaining cell fragments may still be mildly immunogenic. There is no plasma and therefore none of its associated problems. Small amounts of the free haemoglobin, released during processing, probably cause no harm. Hepatitis virus can be transmitted by cryopreserved blood.

Indications for cryopreserved red cells

Frozen red cells are expensive to produce and store; they take one hour to reconstitute and must be used within 12 hours. Their use is therefore limited.

PRESERVATION OF STOCKS OF RARE BLOOD GROUPS

Cryopreservation is the only way of building up useful amounts of red cells of rare blood groups for use in clinical emergencies. For example, persons of blood group KK may develop anti-k (anti-Cellano) antibodies. Since only 2 in 1,000 white people are of KK phenotype, cryopreservation is the best way of ensuring supply.

PREVENTION OF WHITE CELL SENSITIZATION

Frozen red cells are minimally contaminated with white cells (less than 5% of the original white cell count). For individuals in whom HLA immunization must be avoided, such as patients with aplastic anaemia and leukaemia awaiting transplant as well as sensitive patients needing transfusion, they are useful, but filtered blood is usually used for this purpose (page 56).

Red cell products

The currently available red cell products and their characteristics are given in Table 5.2.

Whole blood

The transfusion of whole blood is rarely justified. The only clear indication is for massive haemorrhage when both red cells and volume need to be replaced. In this situation the deleterious effects of high levels of potassium and hydrogen ion, and low levels of active coagulation factors should be minimized by using blood less than five days old.

Plasma reduced blood

Plasma reduced blood and red cells in optimal additive solutions are suitable for general purposes, such as correction of anaemias occurring pre- and post-operatively. Packed red cells may also be used in these situations, although the high haematocrit of 70% or above makes rapid transfusion difficult. They are indicated for patients with chronic anaemias, who are normovolaemic, and commonly in the age group where cardiorespiratory problems occur. The use of packed red cells minimizes fluid overload and pulmonary oedema.

Leucocyte-poor red cells

Leucocyte-poor red cells are indicated for those patients who have developed non-haemolytic, febrile transfusion reactions due to white cell antibodies. Sensitization should be verified by investigation for leukoagglutinins (for granulocytes) or lymphocytotoxic antibodies.

More importantly they are indicated for patients who must avoid sensitization to white cell antigens, particularly HLA antigens, for example patients with aplastic anaemia or leukaemia in remission awaiting bone marrow transplantation. For such patients red cells depleted of over 90% of white cells should be used.

Methods of reducing white cell contamination range from simple centrifugation and removal of the 'buffy-coat' of white cells to machine washing of red cells. Reconstituted frozen red cells, having been washed several times to remove glycerol, contain less than 5% WBC and so can be used as a source of leucocyte depleted blood. The products and their characteristics are shown in Table 5.3.

Microaggregate filters (page 53) used during the transfusion of blood, will remove only 40% of contaminating white cells and are not recommended for this purpose.

Table 5.3 White cell depleted red cells. To prevent white cell related febrile reactions. (*The shelf life of these preparations is either 12 hours if a laminar airflow cabinet is used or 24 hours if a sterile room is used*)

Method	WBC depletion (%)	Red cell loss (%)
Buffy coat poor red cells centrifugation	65–90	10–40
Manually washed buffy coat poor red cells centrifugation and manual washing	90	50
Machine washed red cells centrifugation and automated washing	60–90*	10–40*
White cell poor red cells sedimentation with added dextran or HES	80–95	10
Filtered white cell poor red cells† filtration through cotton or nylon filters	98	10
Frozen red cells† freezing then washing	>95	10

* Depending on whether red cells are already buffy coat poor and the machine used.
† Also used to prevent white cell and HLA sensitization.

White cells are usually removed by wool or nylon filters specifically designed for this purpose (for example Dutch Red Cross or Tyrumo filters). These remove 98% or more of white cells and are very effective in preventing non-haemolytic transfusion reactions as well as sensitization to white cells. These filters are used with blood less than 48 hours old and the procedure is carried out in filtered air cabinets or rooms in the laboratory. Once filtered the red cells have a shelf life of only 24 hours. Such cells are prepared only for specific patients.

Transfusion in acute haemorhage

Acute haemorrhage is a life-threatening situation; rapid clinical evaluation is demanded so that measures to correct hypovolaemia can be instituted. Once resuscitation has been initiated more objective assessment of blood volume and cardiovascular status, such as central venous pressure (CVP), can be made.

The clinical evaluation of blood loss

Initial assessment

GASTROINTESTINAL BLOOD LOSS

Haematemesis usually means blood loss from above the level of the jejunum. The vomiting of fresh unaltered blood indicates *brisk* haemorrhage, possibly from oesophageal varices, and large volumes of blood may be lost rapidly. 'Coffee grounds' altered blood usually arises from the stomach or duodenum and usually represents a slower rate of blood loss.

Melaena does not necessarily originate from the lower intestine. Rapid bleeding from the oesophageal varices or duodenal ulcer eroding the gastroduodenal artery may cause the passage of bright red blood per rectum, because blood is irritant, increasing peristalsis. If the patient has a normal intestinal transit time, the passage of dark red liquid stool usually indicates lesions of the terminal ileum or colon; while black tarry stools indicate bleeding from the upper gastrointestinal tract.

It is obvious that the patient with haematemesis and bright red blood in the stool is in danger of losing a critical blood volume far more rapidly than one with tarry stool only.

The past history may be helpful in deciding the source of the haemorrhage, but it must be remembered that as many as 50% of bleeding episodes in patients with known oesophageal varices are due to other gastrointestinal lesions, and that a patient with a chronic duodenal ulcer can still develop carcinoma of the colon. A patient with known duodenal ulceration who complains of pain radiating to the back and then develops massive haematemesis and melaena may have an erosion of the gastroduodenal artery. However, it has to be remembered that in 20% of patients gastrointestinal bleeding occurs without any previous symptoms.

BLOOD LOSS FROM INJURIES

Clinical assessment of blood lost following injuries sustained during road accidents or other trauma is notoriously difficult. Visible blood loss on to clothing often appears large due to spreading of the bloodstain. Conversely significant amounts of blood may be sequestered in muscle after crush injuries or fractures, without obvious swelling. When swelling is present it can be used as a guide to volume lost, for example, closed tibial fractures with moderate swelling involve blood loss of 500–1,000 ml; femoral fractures with moderate swelling 2,000 ml, with severe swelling 4,000 ml. Pelvic fractures may be associated with over 3,000 ml blood loss.

As an approximate guide to blood loss during open injury to tissues, an area of injury the size of an open hand is taken to represent 500 ml blood loss.

Blood loss into the pleural, peritoneal or pelvic cavities may be missed entirely as little or no swelling may occur even after gross internal haemorrhage. Therefore in any patient with injury to the chest or abdomen internal bleeding should be specifically sought for by examining chest, ribs, diaphragmatic movements, abdominal girth, and assessing peristalsis. Ultrasound is an useful non-invasive investigation. A patient who has hypotension after apparently uncomplicated head injury probably has internal bleeding into the chest or abdomen. Simple head injuries rarely cause hypotension until terminal 'coning' occurs and medullary centres are damaged.

BLOOD LOSS DURING OBSTETRIC ACCIDENTS

Blood loss during obstetric accidents is often very severe, particularly if complicated by disseminated intravascular coagulation or defibrination syndrome associated with sepsis or amniotic fluid embolism. The blood loss is usually obvious and relatively easy to assess but ocasionally, for example, after rupture of the uterus, large volumes may be hidden retroperitoneally before signs of shock draw attention to their occurrence.

Clinical signs of hypovolaema

No matter what the cause of blood loss, nor whether it is obvious or unrecognized, hypovolaemia eventually occurs with its own symptoms and signs, unless there is rapid correction by intravenous therapy.

EARLY SIGNS OF HYPOVOLAEMIA

The 'normal' blood volume is subject to variation. In adults it is 70 ± 10 ml/kg, in neonates it is higher at 85 ml/kg and in the preterm infant is 90 ml/kg. The plasma volume is 45 ± 5 ml/kg; and the red cell volume 30 ± 5 ml/kg in males, 25 ± 5 ml/kg in females. During pregnancy the plasma volume increases from the 10th week, reaching a maximum of around 3,600 ml by the 32nd–34th week. The red cell volume increases more slowly and linearly, so there is a slight fall in haematocrit and haemoglobin during pregnancy.

In some disorders blood volume is altered, for example, during chronic anaemia of any cause the fall in red cell volume is offset by an increase in plasma volume. In splenomegaly the plasma volume rises. In polycythaemia rubra vera the red cell volume rises and, if there is accompanying splenomegaly, the plasma volume will also be raised.

In the previously fit patient loss of 10–15% (around 500 ml) of the initial blood volume is well tolerated. This is because rapid compensation for the decrease in volume is made by sympathetically mediated contraction of the walls of large capacitance veins. This results in a shift of blood into the systemic circulation, so that perfusion of important organs is maintained. There is also a shift of extracellular fluid into the circulation. Blood pressure, cardiac output and oxygen consumption are thus unchanged. Symptoms are transient and mild.

SIGNS OF MODERATELY SEVERE BLOOD LOSS

If blood loss continues until 30% of the volume (around 2 litres) is lost, blood pressure begins to fall and the central and carotid baroreceptors are stimulated, with a resulting increase in sympathetic neuronal discharge. Enhanced production of adrenaline and noradrenaline follows. Adrenaline increases the rate and force of heart muscle contraction with a resultant increase in cardiac output. At the same time the coronary arteries dilate to allow an increased blood supply, whilst arterioles of skin, gut and muscle contract to divert blood to more vital organs. A drop in renal perfusion stimulates the renin angiotensin system with resulting increase in production of aldosterone. This causes sodium and water retention. Antidiuretic hormone is also increased with resultant reduction in urine output. Because of the reduced oxyen supply to some organs anaerobic metabolism will cause an increase in lactic acid production, and compensatory hyperventilation to reduce CO_2 levels and prevent acidosis may occur. Indeed a respiratory alkalosis is common at this stage. The increased cardiac output circulates blood more rapidly and a greater extraction of oxygen may occur with the resultant slight fall in arterial pO_2.

To summarize, the clinical signs of moderate (30% of volume) blood loss are:

(*a*)   Fall in systolic blood pressure below 100 mmHg
(*b*)   Increase in pulse rate above 100/min
(*c*)   Pallor of the skin
(*d*)   Reduced urinary output
(*e*)   Thirst

SIGNS OF SEVERE BLOOD LOSS

As blood loss continues the compensatory mechanisms become inadequate. After 30% or more of the blood volume is lost the blood pressure falls further and there is more intense splanchnic vessel constriction with further reduction in renal blood flow, the blood being diverted to brain and heart muscle only. Anaerobic metabolism is increased, so lactic acidosis progresses and marked compensatory hyperventilation (air hunger) is seen. Eventually, unless successful resuscitation occurs, coronary perfusion falls, the heart muscle fails, consciousness is lost and finally death will occur.

This description of clinical symptoms and signs of hypovolaemia applies to a previously healthy young adult. In the elderly, or those with pre-existing cardiac or respiratory dysfunction the clinical effects of blood loss are accelerated. An elderly person may show all the features of severe haemorrhage after loss of only 20% of his blood volume. Fit young adults may compensate loss of volume so well that they appear unshocked and maintain blood pressure after loss of a relatively

larger volume of blood. Bradycardia may even occur. Any further increment in blood loss can then cause sudden deterioration.

In neonates a very small volume blood loss represents a significant
proportion of the total blood volume. See page 149 for discussion
of blood transfusion in the neonate.

Objective assessment of blood loss and its effects

The clinical history, and examination outlined above can give only
an approximate guide as to the volume of blood loss and its effects.

Once initial measures to stop haemorrhage and replace blood volume
have been taken, and blood samples for full blood count, cross-matching, coagulation screen, biochemical profile and acid/base balance and
blood gas levels have been obtained, objective assessments may be done.

Endoscopy

All cases with significant gastrointestinal haemorrhage should have
urgent endoscopy. This not only allows diagnosis of the causative
lesions, but an assessment of the amount of haemorrhage. Therapeutic
measures such as the injection of varices, mechanical tamponade of
the oesophagus, or laser treatment of bleeding points can also be taken.
Decisions as to the need for emergency surgery can be made.

Measurement of central venous pressure (CVP)

This is necessary in all significant cases of haemorrhage. The central
venous catheter is placed into a central vein and through a three-way
tap can be connected either to an intravenous fluid line or to a manometer.

The fluid level in the manometer is normally 2–10 cm above the
fourth intercostal space in the mid axillary line, but the readings may
be higher if PEEP (Positive End Expiratory Pressure) ventilation is
being used. The central venous presure depends on venous return,
cardiac output and the capacitance of the vascular bed. Tricuspid valve
function also affects the CVP measurement. However, provided left
and right ventricular function are equal the CVP is a useful guide
to fluid replacement. If there is left ventricular dysfunction, this will
eventually cause a rise in CVP and, if it is suspected, measurement
of pulmonary wedge pressure should be undertaken to allow assessment
of left ventricular function separately.

The initial CVP during blood loss is usually low but, if it is over 15 cm H_2O, fluid replacement has been adequate and the rate of infusion should be reduced. A rising CVP suggests either that fluid overload is occurring or 'pump' (heart) failure is developing. A falling CVP may indicate hypovolaemia or deteriorating cardiac function.

A useful test during the management of hypovolaemia is the fluid challenge test. The CVP is noted and then 200 ml of dextran 70 (page 191) is infused over 15 minutes. The CVP is then noted immediately, and after 10 minutes.

(*a*)   If the CVP fails to rise, there is no danger of fluid overload and replacement may continue.

(*b*)   If it rises by 5 cm but then falls to the initial value at 10 minutes, fluid overload is still unlikely and cautious replacement can proceed.

(*c*)   If the CVP rises by over 5 cm and remains elevated at 10 minutes, the i.v. infusion rate must be reduced.

Blood loss during surgery

In order that blood lost during surgery can be promptly replaced patients are grouped and screened for antibodies or blood is cross-matched depending on the operation (Table 5.4).

The assessment of blood loss during surgical operations is made difficult by several factors. The amount of blood lost cannot easily be assessed in severe cases because loss on to drapes, surgeons' gowns and even the floor cannot be measured. The patient's response to hypovolaemia, a useful clinical guide to the severity of blood loss, is interfered with by anaesthetic drugs. Hypotension may be due to vasodilation caused by drugs, or vasovagal responses, rather than blood loss. Sophisticated techniques such as colorimetric estimation of haemoglobin washed from swabs, or continuous patient weighing are laborious and time-consuming and still subject to error. For these reasons, simple guidelines that allow an approximate estimate of blood loss have been evolved.

In all cases the task of monitoring blood loss and charting intravenous replacement should be delegated to a single member of the surgical team.

Blood loss into suction bottles is relatively easy to measure. Small diameter vessels give more accurate volume readings than larger ones. Weighing the vessel before and after filling will allow a more accurate

Table 5.4   Transfusion guidelines for elective surgery

General surgery
Cholecystectomy	Group and screen
Exploratory laparotomy	Group and screen
Hiatus hernia repair	Group and screen
Colectomy and hemicolectomy	2 units
Splenectomy	2 units
Breast biopsy	Group and screen
Mastectomy	1 unit
Gastrectomy	2 units
Antrectomy and vagotomy	2 units
Inguinal herniorrhaphy	Group and screen
Vein stripping	Group and screen

Cardiovascular surgery
Saphenous vein bypass	8 units
Congenital open heart surgery	8 units
Valve replacement	8 units
Aortobifemoral bypass	8 units
Thoracotomy	3 units
Closed mediastinal exploration	Group and screen
Resection abdominal aortic aneurysm	8 units
Carotid endarterectomy	2 units

Obstetric-gynaecologic surgery
Total abdominal hysterectomy	Group and screen
Exploratory laparotomy	Group and screen
Total vaginal hysterectomy	Group and screen
Laparoscopy	Group and screen
Repeat caesarian section	Group and screen
Labour and delivery requests	Group and screen

Plastic surgery
Mammoplasty	Group and screen
Thoracoabdominal flap	Group and screen

Orthopaedic surgery
Open reduction	2 units
Arthroplasty	Group and screen
Shoulder reconstruction	Group and screen
Total hip replacement	2–3 units
Total knee replacement	Group and screen

Genitourinary surgery
Transurethral resection of prostate	Group and screen
Radical nephrectomy	1 unit
Renal transplantation	1 unit
Prostatectomy	2 units

Modified from Boral, L I *et al* (1979) *American Journal of Clinical Pathology* **71**, 680–684 calculation of blood loss, particularly if frothing makes volume readings difficult. Large volumes of ascitic or amniotic fluid diluting the blood should be taken into account.

Swabs (of known standard weight) should be weighed after use; each gram of weight gain represents approximately 1 ml of blood loss. Swabs can be weighed in batches of five to save time. The time elapsing between swab use and weighing must be minimized, otherwise loss of weight will occur due to evaporation. During blood loss in neonates and children, swabs must be weighed singly. Some surgeons prefer to use moistened swabs. The volume of fluid used for this should be monitored and subtracted from the estimate of blood loss. It is usually found that swab weighing and suction-bottle volume measurements lead to an underestimate of blood loss. There is often hidden loss within the body cavities, in traumatized tissue and ligatured vessels. During orthopaedic surgery blood is sequestered in muscles and bone cavities.

For these reasons, when major surgery likely to involve massive blood loss is planned, special measures are taken to enable better assessment of hypovolaemia and its effects. A central venous pressure (CVP) line is inserted preoperatively so that a baseline level is available, and any changes can be interpreted meaningfully (page 62). A urinary catheter is put in and urinary output, reflecting renal perfusion, is monitored. The minimum urine flow should be 0.5 ml/kg/h (around 30–35 ml/h).

Heat sensitive electrodes are used for assessment of skin:core temperature difference. Usually the electrodes are placed on a digit (great toe) and in the external auditory meatus. If there is adequate perfusion, the readings should be identical. If there is a difference of over 2°C, tissue perfusion is inadequate and corrective measures are needed.

The management of acute haemorrhage

Blood should be taken for cross-matching, baseline haemoglobin and haematocrit, and coagulation screen. Intravenous access is established and volume is maintained using crystalloids such as normal saline or colloids such as the synthetic plasma expanders (page 191) or albumin (page 111). During early haemorrhage maintenance of the plasma volume and the circulation is critical because there is a good reserve in the oxygen carrying capacity of haemoglobin. In normal individuals the amount of oxygen available from haemoglobin is four times basal needs. During severe haemorrhage more of the oxygen carried by haemoglobin becomes available as the oxygen dissociation curve shifts to the right because of the accumulation of lactic and pyruvic acid.

Provided the plasma volume can be maintained the increased cardiac output will ensure adequate oxygen delivery to the tissues until blood becomes available.

Choice of volume replacement fluid

Crystalloids are non-allergenic, cheap and easy to obtain. However, if large volumes are used, they may reduce the plasma colloid oncotic pressure and cause interstitial fluid to accumulate. Pulmonary oedema may develop. This is not always signalled by a rise in the CVP as the fluid disappears rapidly into the extracellular space where it does not affect the CVP.

Colloids such as albumin, having larger molecules, are less likely to leak out of the vessels. They are therefore osmotically more active and less likely to cause pulmonary oedema. Rarely albumin and plasma protein fraction may contain prekallikrein activators which cause hypotension. Dextran and other non-human colloids may cause allergic reactions, impaired coagulation and renal toxicity. Rarely they may make subsequent cross-matching of blood difficult. The use and properties of the volume expanders are discussed in Chapter 13.

Having resuscitated the patient using volume replacement fluids, blood transfusion is begun. In massive haemorrhage whole blood, preferably less than four days old, is indicated. This has the advantage that the coagulation factors are more active, there has been minimal accumulation of hydrogen and potassium ions in the plasma and there is maximum red cell viability. Neonates should always be given fresh blood (page 150).

In less brisk haemorrhage plasma-reduced or packed cells may be used, supplemented by fresh frozen plasma to replace coagulation factors if necessary.

In all cases when 10 or more units of stored blood have been transfused the coagulation function and platelet count should be assessed and replacement given if indicated (page 70). The elderly and those with hepatic impairment are likely to require such replacement earlier.

Transfusion of over 4 units of blood involves the risk of the accumulation of microaggregates. Standard blood filters (170 μm) will not remove these and microaggregate filters (20–40 μm) should be used. Platelets are best given through the standard filter, as they are impeded by microaggregate filters. When large volumes are to be used blood should be transfused through a blood warmer to prevent hypothermia. Calcium replacement may also be necessary because of the citrate used (page 70).

Transfusion in chronic anaemias

During the development of chronic anaemia, when the red cell volume falls slowly, there is time for adaptive mechanisms which increase oxygen delivery to the tissues, to occur. The two main mechanisms are:

(*a*)   Reduction in the oxygen affinity of the haemoglobin by an increase in red cell 2,3DPG.

(*b*)   Increase in cardiac output, so that the rate of oxygen delivery to the tissues increases.

Reduction in the activity of the individual concerned also conserves oxygen.

Changes in 2,3DPG

As anaemia develops 2,3DPG rises in the red cells and reduces haemoglobin oxygen affinity. This is brought about by two mechanisms. In the first it binds to the deoxy- or low affinity form of haemoglobin, altering the equilibrium between its high and low affinity states reducing the oxygen affinity. The second is due to a fall of intracellular pH caused by the increase of 2,3DPG. This results in a shift of the oxygen dissociation curve to the right, causing an increased proportion of oxygen to be released at a given tissue pO_2. There is also a small fall in the mean venous pO_2 further increasing oxygen release. These changes can increase oxygen release by up to 50%. For example, an individual with a haemoglobin of 6g/dl can release the same amount as an individual with a haemoglobin of 9g/dl with the oxygen dissociation curve at the normal position. These changes are at the expense of the oxygen reserve in the blood, and the ability to compensate for exercise is reduced.

It is because of these adaptive mechanisms that chronic anaemia in an otherwise healthy individual rarely causes symptoms until the haemoglobin falls below 10g/dl.

Changes in cardiac output

As the haemoglobin falls below 10g/dl there is a rise, first in the stroke volume and then in cardiac rate, increasing cardiac output and oxygen delivery to the tissues. However, the cardiac reserve is reduced and further demand on exertion cannot be met. The symptoms of severe anaemia (Hb less than 5g/dl) therefore include palpitations, breathlessness on exertion and, in those with pre-existing cardiac dysfunction, oedema.

Transfusion in the treatment of chronic anaemias

The decision to restore haemoglobin levels by transfusion in patients with chronic anaemia should not be taken lightly. Transfusion has a mortality and this is greater in the elderly and in those with cardiac dysfunction. Those with chronic anaemias often fall within these categories and in addition they have an increased plasma volume in compensation for their reduced red cell volume.

If the anaemia can be treated by other means these should be considered first. For example in iron, Vitamin B_{12} or folate deficiency the haemoglobin will rise by one gram per week if the appropriate haematinic is given. Therefore, unless the anaemia is disabling at rest or there is another reason for restoring the haemoglobin level quickly, such as imminent delivery or urgent surgery, transfusion is best avoided. Transfusion can be fatal in severely anaemic, elderly patients.

For urgent operations a haemoglobin level of at least 10g/dl is recommended, although this level may be a little generous in patients with normal cardiorespiratory function in view of the compensatory changes in red cell oxygen delivery.

In patients in whom surgery is not urgent, and the anaemia is remediable, treatment with haematinics is to be preferred to the expediency of a 'quick transfusion'. Single unit transfusions are unnecessary.

In patients with chronic unremediable anaemia such as aplastic anaemia, myelodysplastic syndromes and the leukaemias transfusion is the only way to maintain haemoglobin levels. In such patients it may not be necessary to transfuse to a 'normal' haemoglobin level because of the adaptive mechanisms noted above. In most persons a level of around 10g/dl is sufficient to maintain oxygenation and relieve the symptoms of anaemia.

Clinical practice

(*a*) Patients with chronic anaemias should be transfused with 'packed cells' as they already have a raised plasma volume.

(*b*) In the elderly or those with cardiorespiratory disease transfusion should be preceded by an i.v. injection of 40 mg frusemide, and further 20 mg doses should be given with alternate units to avoid volume overload.

(*c*) In the severely anaemic, elderly patient transfusion should be given in *separate* amounts, e.g. 2 units over 8 hours on the first day, and repeated 24 to 48 hours later if necessary. Again frusemide should be given. The drip should be taken down between transfusions to avoid volume overload by the infusion of saline.

The special problems of transfusion in thalassaemia major and sickle cell disease are discussed below.

Transfusion in specific diseases

Sickle cell disease

Sickle cell disease in this context means any of the sickling syndromes which give rise to haemolysis, i.e. homozygous sickle cell disease, sickle cell Hb-C disease, sickle cell β-thalassaemia, etc., but not sickle cell trait. Transfusion in sickle cell disease is not indicated for anaemia but is useful for terminating crises, preparing patients for major surgery and prophylaxis against crises during pregnancy. If possible, exchange transfusion should be used to prevent eventual iron overload.

In these multiply transfused patients blood group and white cell antibodies often occur and Rh and Kell genotyped matched filtered blood is used.

TRANSFUSION DURING CRISES

This is not indicated as a routine but may be used in a prolonged, exceptionally severe crisis. It is indicated for certain complications. These are: chest complications (sickle lung syndrome), suspicion of central nervous system involvement, septicaemia or severe local infection, for example, osteomyelitis. In these patients a partial exchange transfusion should be carried out. Blood containing sickled cells has a higher than normal viscosity and the anaemia partly protects the patients from some of its effects. The aim of the exchange transfusion therefore should be to keep the haemoglobin at the patients usual level until there are more than 50% normal red cells in his blood. This is particularly important in some of the sickle cell syndromes, such as sickle cell haemoglobin C disease, which can have a normal haemoglobin level.

PREPARATION OF PATIENTS FOR SURGERY

The patient's sickle red cells are replaced with normal red cells and more than 70% Hb-A red cells should be aimed for; this is indicated for all except very minor operations particularly if hypoxia is expected. This is best done by exchange tranfusion. To reach the required level it may have to be done twice with a few days interval.

PROPHYLACTIC TRANSFUSION DURING PREGNANCY

Although there are no data to indicate that prophylactic transfusion during pregnancy reduces the incidence of sickle complications, this is often done at 28 weeks of pregnancy and is carried out using 4 units of packed cells. The patient is then transfused at weekly or fortnightly intervals with 2 to 3 units of packed cells until the Hb-A cells exceed 70% of total cells. As sickle cells have a short survival this is not difficult to achieve. If the patient has a sickle crisis before the 28th week, the transfusion programme is started at that time.

β-thalassaemia major

Once it has been decided on clinical grounds, such as failure to thrive, the development of cardiac failure and a low haemoglobin that a patient has thalassaemia major (and not thalassaemia intermedia), he is put on a transfusion regime to maintain a haemoglobin level of at least 9g/dl. With such a regime children are active and grow normally but still have considerable marrow activity, most of which is ineffective, and a minimum level of haemoglobin of 11g/dl is now recommended. This higher level is particularly indicated if there is considerable iron overload with cardiac involvement. As these patients are at risk for the development of white cell antibodies filtered blood should be used to prevent sensitization or reaction. The amount of blood given to a 50 kg adult would be 3 units every four to five weeks. The pre- and post-transfusion haemoglobin levels and volumes of blood transfused are carefully documented. These are used to determine the rate of haemoglobin fall and the amount of blood used. If these become excessive, a rate of haemoglobin fall greater than 1% of total haemoglobin per day or more than 230 ml 70% packed cells transfused per kg body weight per year, splenectomy for hypersplenism is indicated. Such figures can only be worked out over a minimum period of six months.

Recently the use of 'young red cells' has been tried in order to reduce the rate of iron loading and lengthen the transfusion interval. The results show that any gain is marginal and this is no longer used. Another approach suggested has been to partially exchange transfuse the patient, removing a proportion of the senescent red cell population and consequently reducing iron loading.

Patients with thalassaemia intermedia should not be regularly transfused as iron chelation therapy is not adequate at the present time (page 147).

Paroxysmal nocturnal haemoglobinuria

Plasma may supply factors (complement) which may increase haemolysis and washed, filtered red cells should be used.

Massive transfusions

Massive transfusions are needed during cardiac surgery, for obstetric complications and to combat uncontrolled bleeding. Special measures are necessary if more than three-quarters of the patient's blood volume has been replaced.

Haemostasis

Thrombocytopenia: this can become severe, platelet concentrates should be given according to the count or one pack with every 4 units after the first 6.

Coagulation defects: These are due mainly to a fall in factors V and VIII and occur after 6–10 units have been transfused. Therapy with FFP should be controlled by results of the prothrombin and partial thromboplastin time. Alternatively one pack of FFP can be given with every 4 units after the first 6.

Metabolic effects

These are mixed; the relative acidity of the blood may cause a metabolic acidosis, whereas the citrate in the anticoagulant may cause a metabolic alkalosis. Occasionally a high plasma potassium can occur, but usually cellular metabolism will reduce this quickly. Ionized calcium may fall due to the citrate in the stored blood, particularly if the transfusion is given rapidly, and tetany and cardiac arrhythmia may result. The effect of citrate is bigger if there is impairment of liver function. Treatment is with 10 ml of 10% calcium gluconate i.v. with every litre of blood transfused rapidly.

Oxygen affinity

Stored blood has a high oxygen affinity due to a fall in the 2,3DPG in the red cells (page 48). If massive transfusions are to be given, relatively fresh blood, less than five days old, should be given.

Management of masssive transfusions requires ECG and central venous pressure monitoring on one hand, with coagulation studies, platelet counts, haemoglobin, calcium, potassium and blood gas measurements by the laboratory. Speed is very important and special arrangements for measurements on such patients are essential. Abnormalities of haemostasis call for the appropriate replacement with fresh frozen plasma and platelets. Prophylactic administration is outlined above. A fall in the central venous pressure may indicate a failure of blood replacement to match blood loss and should be treated appropriately.

Further reading

Dawson, R B (1983) Preservation of red blood cells for transfusion. *Human Pathology*, **14**, 213–217.

Collins, J A (1983) Pertinent recent developments in blood banking. *Surgical Clinics of North America*, **63**, 483–485.

Hogman, C F, Hedlund, K, Zetterström, H (1978) Clinical usefulness of red cells preserved in protein poor mediums. *New England Journal of Medicine*, **299**, 1377–1382.

Heaton, A, Miripol, J, Aster, R, Hartmann, P, Dehart, D, Rzadl, B, Grapka, A W, Davisson, W, Buchholz, D (1984) Use of Adsol preservation solution for prolonged storage of low viscosity AS-1 red blood cells. *British Journal of Haematology*, **57**, 467–478.

Valeri, C R, Valeri, D A, Gray, A, Melaragno, A, Dennis, R C, Emerson, C P (1982) Viability and function of red blood cell concentrates stored at 4°C for 35 days in CPDA-1, CPDA-2, or CPDA-3. *Transfusion*, **22**, 210–216.

International Forum (1978) What is the toxicological importance of the liberation of pthalates from plastic containers into blood, its components and derivatives? *Vox Sanguinis*, **34**, 244–254.

Gilcher, R O (1982) Blood and apheresis products: usage in modern transfusion therapy. *Plasma Therapy*, **3**, 27–44.

Hughes, A S, Brozovic, B (1982) Leucocyte depleted blood: an appraisal of available techniques. *British Journal of Haematology*, **50**, 381–386.

Boral, L I, Dannemiller, F J, Stanford, W, Hill, S S, Cornell, T A (1978)

A guideline for anticipated blood usage during elective surgical procedures. *American Journal of Clinical Pathology*, **71**, 680–684.

Rush, B F (1974) Volume replacement: when, what and how much? In: *Treatment of Shock: Principles and Practice*. Eds. Schumer, W, Nyhus, L M. Lea and Febiger, Philadelphia.

6 Platelet concentrates

Platelet function in fresh whole blood starts to decline rapidly six hours after collection, and the numbers of platelets present in a single unit are too small for therapeutic use. Therefore, for platelet replacement concentrates are prepared from blood obtained from several donors or by plateletpheresis of a single donor. Such concentrates became generally available for use in thrombocytopenia in the early 1960s. Their value is illustrated by the fact that death from haemorrhage in acute leukaemia dropped from over 60% to 15% between 1960 and 1966.

Structure and function of platelets

Platelets are non-nucleated, discoid structures 2–4 μm in diameter, whose shape is maintained by a circumferential system of microtubules (Fig. 6.1).

The function of platelets is to maintain primary haemostasis. Normally, provided vascular endothelium is intact, platelets remain inert. If the endothelium is breached, microfibrils and collagen, to which platelets rapidly adhere, are exposed. This adherence is mediated by a specific platelet surface receptor and the plasma factor VIIIVWF. If the specific platelet receptor is missing (as in the congenital disorder Bernard Soulier disease) or the plasma factor is missing (as in von Willebrand's disease), platelet adhesion will be defective. Intact endothelium secretes prostaglandin I_2 (PGI_2) a potent agent which prevents inappropriate adhesion of pre-activated platelets to the endothelium. Platelet adhesion is enhanced by high shear rates within blood vessels and by the presence of thrombin.

Having adhered to the injured vessel wall, platelets undergo the release reaction, which *in vitro* is preceded by a change in platelet shape and granule distribution, with the appearance of pseudopods. During

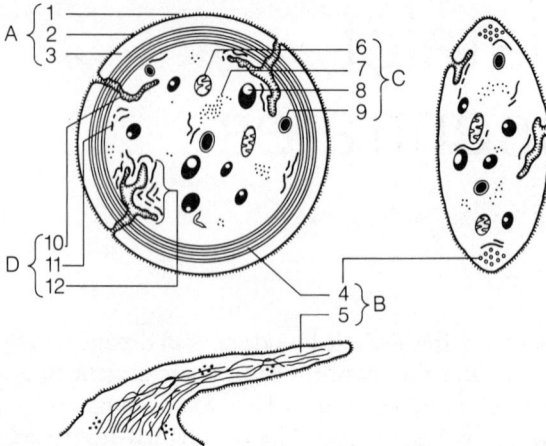

Fig. 6.1 Morphology of non-activated platelets. The ultrastructural features observed in non-activated platelets, cut in the equatorial plane (*top left*) and in cross section (*top right*), as well as in a pseudopod of an activated platelet (*bottom*). The peripheral zone (A) consists of the glycocalyx (1), the trilaminar unit membrane (2) and the submembrane area (3). The sol-gel zone (B) consists of the microtubules (4) and the microfilaments which become detectable during activation (5). The organelle zone (C) contains, *inter alia*, mitochondria (6), glycogen (7), α-granules (8) and dense bodies (9). The membrane systems (D) consists of the open canalicular system (10), the dense tubular system (11) and the membrane complexes (12). (From Vermylen, J et al (1983) Normal mechanisms of platelet function, *Clinics in Haematology*, **12,** 108)

release the contents of the platelet granules are discharged. The main substances released and their function is shown in Table 6.1.

Table 6.1   Major substances liberated during platelet release

Substance	Function
ADP	Induces platelet aggegation
5HT	Vasoconstriction and increased vascular permeability
Calcium	Promotes coagulation
Prostaglandins Thromboxane A2	Induce further platelet release and aggregation
Platelet factor 4	Neutralizes heparin
Thromboglobulin	Inhibits PGI_2 production
Platelet-derived growth factor	Stimulates smooth muscle and fibroblast growth
Antiplasmin	Inhibits fibrinolysis

Released substances, especially ADP and thromboxane A_2 cause the platelets to aggregate and induce new platelets to undergo the release and aggregation process, amplifying the response. If the original stimulus was relatively weak, aggregation is reversible. Stronger stimuli activate the metabolism of a platelet-membrane-bound substance, arachidonic acid, with the production of further thromboxane A_2 and prostaglandins (Fig. 6.2), resulting in irreversible aggregation.

Once a firm plug of aggregated platelets has formed, whole blood coagulation is promoted and fibrin is formed. The property of activated platelets in promoting whole blood coagulation is known as platelet factor III activity. The interactions of activated factor IX and X are particularly enhanced. The phenomena involved in platelet aggregation are outlined in Fig. 6.3.

In the laboratory, platelet function is assessed using platelet-rich plasma separated from the patient's citrated blood. Adhesion can be assessed by the degree of retention of platelets occurring when a sample is passed over a column of glass beads. Aggregation is assessed by the changes in adsorption of a beam of light by a sample of platelets exposed to aggregating agents such as collagen, ADP or ristocetin under controlled conditions. An example of a normal platelet aggregation curve and its relationship to phenomena observed during aggregation is shown in Fig. 6.4.

The platelet specific antigens are described in Chapter 3, and HLA antigens on platelets in Chapter 4.

Collection of platelets

Platelet donors should not have been taking any anti-platelet drugs, such as aspirin for 14 days before donation.

Standard blood donations

During donor sessions a planned number of donations is collected into special 'triple' or 'quadruple' closed system packs which are designed to facilitate subsequent harvest of platelets (Fig. 5.2). Within six hours of collection these packs are centrifuged at 1,000 × **g** for 10 minutes, and the resultant platelet-rich plasma is extruded by pressure into a satellite pack within the closed system. This is centrifuged at 3,000 × **g** for 20 minutes after which the bulk of the plasma is removed achieving a concentrate containing 85% of the platelets of

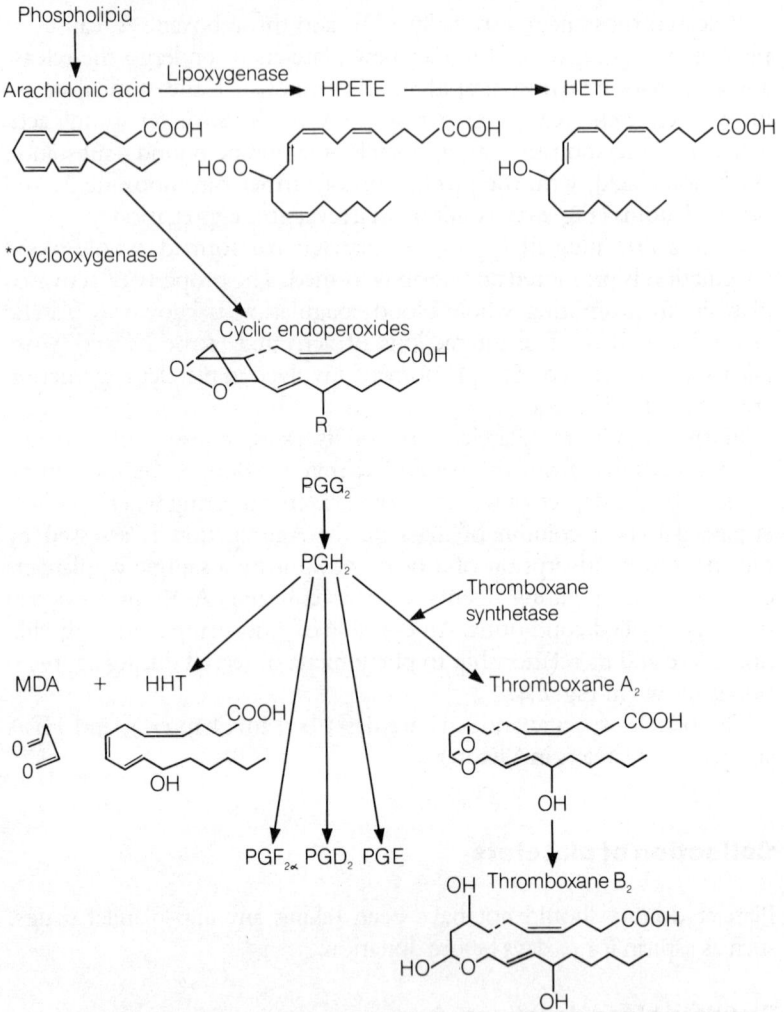

Fig. 6.2 Pathways of arachidonic-acid metabolism in human platelets. HPETE, 12-hydroperoxy-eicosatetraenoic acid; HETE, 12-hydroxy-eicosatetraenoic acid; MDA, malonyl dialdehyde; HHT, 12-hydroxy-hepatadecatrienoic acid. *Point of action of aspirin and indomethacin. (From Hardisty, R M and Weatherall, D J (1982), *Blood and its Disorders*, Blackwell, Oxford)

the original donation. These are resuspended in 50–70 ml of residual plasma, to achieve a final concentration of not more than $1.7 \times 10^{12}/l$. The total number of platelets in each pack is about 0.5×10^{11}. Six such packs are used for each platelet transfusion.

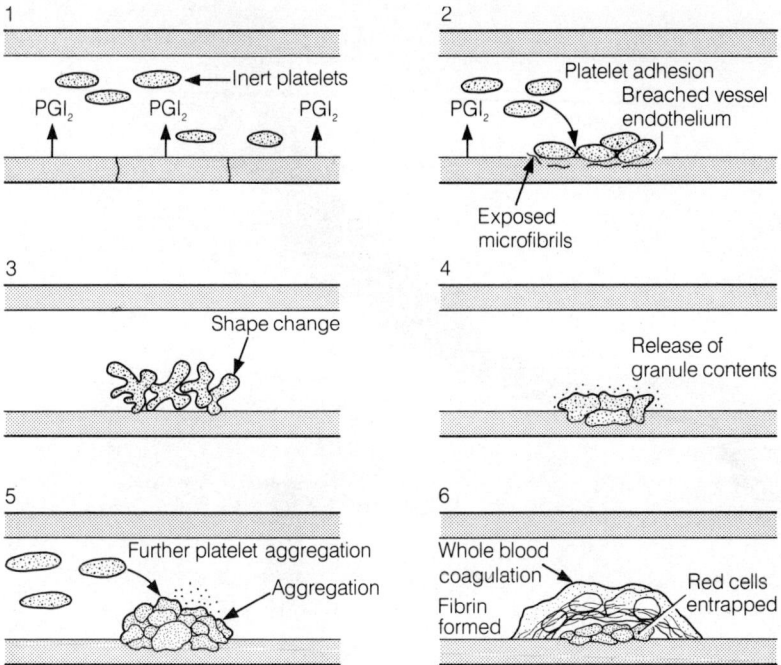

Fig. 6.3 The formation of a thrombus in a blood vessel.

Plateletpheresis

Plateletpheresis can be carried out using either a continuous or intermittent type of cell separator (Chapter 12). With such systems up to $2-5 \times 10^{11}$ platelets can be collected at one time. This is particularly useful for the supply of single donor platelets to individuals sensitized to HLA or platelet specific antigens, but are also used for the general supply of platelets. Platelet concentrates prepared by plateletpheresis involving an 'open' procedure must be used within 24 hours of preparation, to minimize multiplication of any contaminating organisms.

Quality assessment of platelet concentrates

Platelets have a tendency to aggregate in response to minimal trauma such as collision together during the preparation process. This causes damage and reduces subsequent viability and function. Because of this,

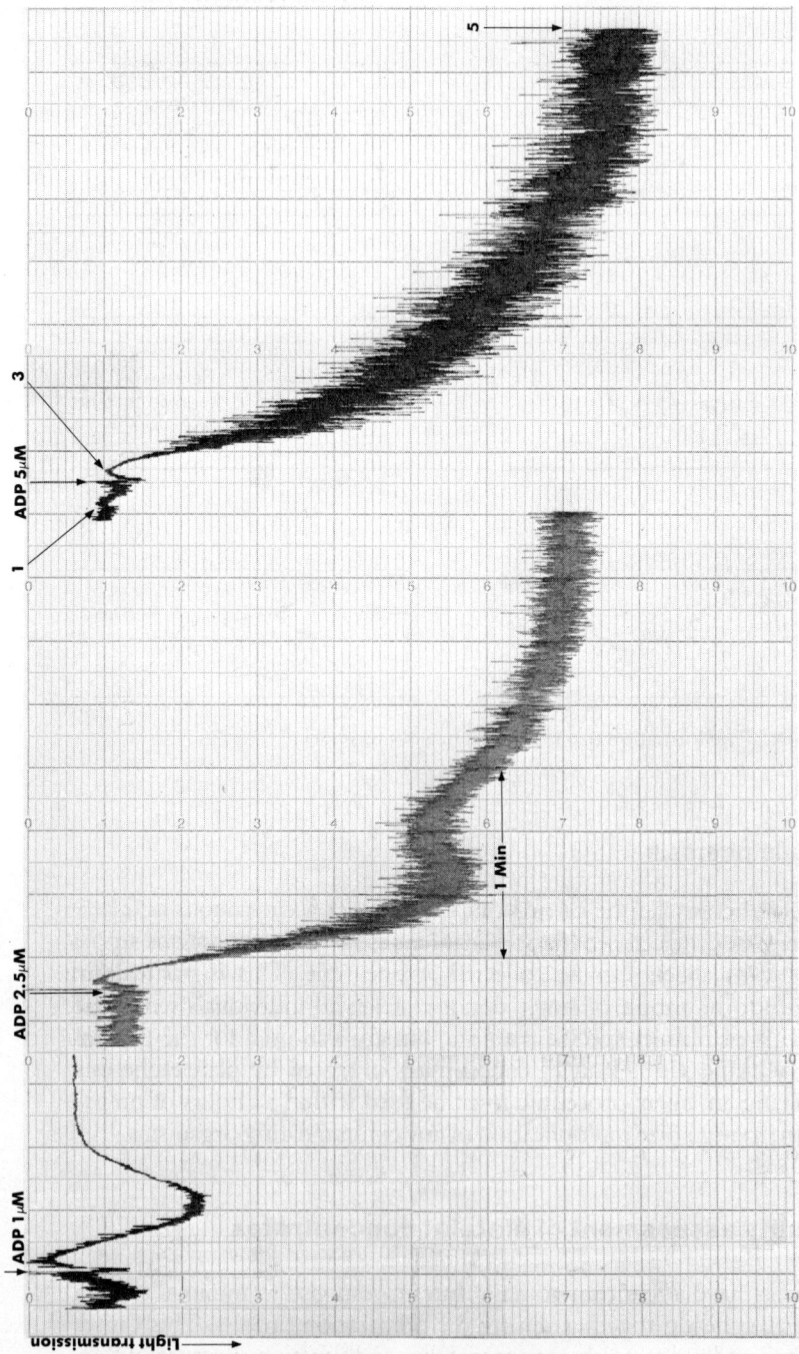

Fig. 6.4 Platelet shape change and aggregation in response to ADP: 1 μm, first phase only; 2.5 μm, biphasic; 5 μm irreversible aggregation. Numbers 1, 3 and 5 refer to Fig. 6.3.

methods of platelet production and storage have to be rigorously evaluated and controlled.

Platelet recovery, survival and viability

The recovery, survival and viability of stored platelets after infusion can be compared with that of fresh autologous platelets, the latter being used to avoid the complication of immune destruction.

The platelets are labelled with either [111]indium or ^{51}Cr neither of which are reused during thrombopoiesis. The bound radioactivity is then counted and the platelets are infused. Blood samples are taken immediately and at intervals over the first hour and then daily for six days. The platelet radioactivity in the samples is then plotted against time.

Platelet survival curves show that fresh autologous platelets have a life span of approximately nine days. There is an initial fall in radioactivity during the first ten minutes after injection, due to splenic sequestration of about one-third of platelets. With massive splenomegaly this is larger and equilibration may take up to 60 minutes.

$$\text{Platelet recovery} = \frac{\text{Platelet 'counts' at time zero} \times \text{blood volume}}{\text{Total platelet activity injected}}$$

Normal recovery = 50–70% for fesh platelets

Viability is a function of initial recovery and survival, and can be expressed as the area measured under the survival curve. The value obtained for stored platelets can be compared with that for fresh platelets and expressed as a percentage.

Template bleeding time correction

The effects of infusion of fresh ABO and Rh compatible platelets on platelet increment and bleeding time of a population of thrombocytopenic patients is recorded. The effects of stored compatible platelets is then compared. Provided platelet function is normal, bleeding time and platelet count are inversely related. Although theoretically the best test of platelet efficacy, bleeding time studies on thrombocytopenic cases are difficult to standardize and compare.

Since many factors affect the increment and function achieved by platelet transfusions the patients used for these tests must:

1   have thrombocytopenia due to marrow failure,
2   be free of platelet antibodies,
3   have no splenomegaly,
4   be afebrile,
5   not be bleeding.

Platelet adhesion

Platelet adhesion to glass beads or damaged animal aortic tissue is assessed for fresh normal platelets and for stored concentrate platelets.

Platelet aggregation

Samples of fresh normal platelets and sorted platelets are subjected, under controlled conditions, to the effects of the common aggregating agents, thrombin, ADP and collagen. Fig 6.4

Hypotonic shock response

This measures the ability of platelets to regain their normal discoid shape after rapid sphering in hypotonic solution and reflects their metabolic integrity. As in platelet aggregation studies the change in transmission of a beam of light is used to indicate the change in shape of platelets on addition of distilled water. The response of stored platelets is expressed as a percentage of that of fresh platelets.

pH

The pH of stored platelets is one of the simplest quality control measurements, and is particularly important for platelets stored at 22°C and should not fall below 6.0.

Metabolic parameters

These are of greatest relevance when platelets are stored at 22°C. They include measurements of:

Lactate
ATP/ADP
Glycolytic intermediates
Glycolytic enzymes
pO_2, pCO_2
Platelet factor 3 availability

Serotonin uptake (5HT)

Viable platelets take up 5HT actively against a concentration gradient. Under controlled conditions measurement of uptake of 5HT is said to evaluate energy metabolism and integrity of the plasma membrane.

Ultrastructural changes

Normal platelets are discoid. The most constant feature predicting poor *in-vivo* viability is a permanent change in shape from discs to spheres. This occurs at extremes of pH (below 6 and over 7.4), immediately on cooling to 4°C and more slowly during storage at 22°C.

Purity of the concentrate

The extent to which erythrocytes and leucocytes contaminate concentrates produced by different methods can be compared.

Bacterial contamination

Any new procedure for collection or storage must be assessed for the risks of bacterial contamination. Procedures involving systems 'open' to the atmosphere such as some plateletpheresis procedures are more likely to be contaminated.

Characteristics of various platelet concentrates

The quality of currently available platelet concentrates in terms of *in-vitro* and *in-vivo* performance is outlined below according to variables that have been identified as important.

Collection variables

Platelets prepared from standard donations are frequently contaminated by red cells, and contain up to 20% of the leucocytes of the original donation. Centrifugal forces used during preparation consistently impair platelet adhesiveness and the **g** force must be kept below 3,000 to prevent greater injury resulting in reduced viability.

Platelets prepared by platelet-pheresis undergo lower **g** forces but still have reduced adhesiveness. Provided centrifugal forces do not exceed 3,000 × **g** there is no difference in viability before storage between standard and machine produced platelet concentrates.

Storage variables

The temperature at which platelets are stored is the single most important variable since it determines metabolic activity of the cells, and temperature effects may also directly damage them. Table 6.2 shows the characteristics of platelets stored at 4°C and 22°C.

Table 6.2   Characteristics of platelets stored at stated temperature in ACD

Temperature (°C)	Storage time (hours)	Recovery (%)	Survival (days)
	fresh	55	8
4	24	60	1
4	72	40	1
22	24	50	8
22	72	40	8
22	96	25	4

(Adapted from Slichter, S J (1970), *British Journal of Haematology*, **34**, 403)

Storage at 4°C

Concentrates at this temperature are metabolically inactive, and measurements reflecting metabolic activity remain static.

In-vitro tests of aggregation function show good responses, and immediate post-transfusion recovery *in vivo* is comparable with platelets stored at 22°C. However, it has been shown that cold injures the platelet circumferential microtubular system, resulting in a permanent shape change from discs to spheres. This is correlated with a poor post-transfusion survival *in vivo*. The beneficial effects of 4°C stored platelets on the bleeding time of thrombocytopenic patients is thus short lived, lasting only 24 hours. The only advantage of 4°C storage is that bacterial contaminants will fail to multlpy.

Storage at 22°C

Recovery and survival of platelets after storage at 22°C is superior to that of platelets stored in the cold. However, platelets stored at this temperature retain their metabolic activity. They metabolize glucose, consume oxygen and produce carbon dioxide and lactic acid. If oxygen is depleted, anaerobic glycolysis produces further lactic acid and the pH falls. CO_2 accumulation exacerbates the pH fall. As the pH falls below 6 a permanent shape change from discs to spheres occurs in the platelets, as the circumferential microtubular system is damaged. A similar change occurs if the pH is allowed to rise above 7.4.

As with platelets stored at 4°C the damage to the circumferential microtubular system is correlated with poor survival after infusion. In order to maintain pH between 6 and 7.4 the following have been adopted:

1   Resuspension of platelets in 50–70 ml of residual plasma which provides buffering capacity. Platelet concentration must not be above $1.7 \times 10^{12}/l$.
2   Use of thin-walled, relatively large volume storage bags, with flatbed agitation, to promote entry of oxygen and release of CO_2. Polyolefin plastics, e.g. Fenwal PL732 with high gas permeability have been developed for this purpose.
3   Use of CPD based anticoagulant which is of higher pH than ACD.

Despite the relatively good survival times *in vivo*, function of platelets stored at 22°C is not entirely normal. Aggregation studies show reduced function in comparison with platelets stored at 4°C. However, it has been reported that this function is rapidly restored once the platelets are infused. The hypotonic shock response shows that platelets stored at 22°C recover better from hypotonic stress than those stored at 4°C and this correlates well with the survival of platelets stored at 22°C.

Measurements of metabolic parameters reflect the fact that platelets stored at 22°C remain metabolically active, retaining capacity for glycolysis, serotonin uptake, oxygen consumption and CO_2 release. The superior clinical effectiveness of platelets stored at 22°C is shown by the fact that they reduce bleeding times in thrombocytopenic patients, even after 72 hours storage. The effect is also more lasting.

It has been suggested that the superior performance of 4°C stored platelets in terms of aggregation function, and the increased viability of platelets stored at 22°C could be combined by 'cycling' the temperature of platelets during storage. For example, platelets stored at 4°C could be subjected to 12-hourly periods at 37°C of 30 minutes duration.

Cryopreservation of platelets

Effective cryopreservation of platelets would enable large stocks to be built up, and allow planned storage of autologous platelets obtained by plateletpheresis. The latter would be indicated for patients in remission from acute leukaemia awaiting bone marrow transplantation. Unfortunately freezing damages living cells, and low-temperature storage is expensive. Cryopreserved platelets are therefore not widely available. If freezing occurs too rapidly, intracellular ice crystals form, and integrity is lost. At slower rates of freezing the ice crystals tend to form extracellularly, effectively concentrating the residual solution and causing osmotic damage. For those reasons the rate of freezing must be carefully controlled and a cryoprotectant such as dimethylsulphoxide (DMSO) or glycerol is required. DMSO is the most commonly used cryoprotectant for platelet preservation. It is added to a final concentration of 4–6% to the platelets, which are then frozen in polyolefin bags at a rate of 0.5–10°C per minute. The resulting platelets can be stored in liquid nitrogen or a mechanical freezer at −80°C for up to three years. Because DMSO is toxic the platelets must be washed prior to infusion, and resuspended in plasma or balanced salt solution.

The quality of the recovered platelets is assessed by the methods previously outlined. The immediate post-transfusion recovery is 65–70%. The survival is around 30% of that expected from fresh platelets, and is in general inferior to platelets stored at 22°C. Although they shorten the bleeding time in thrombocytopenic patients, their performance *in vitro* during aggregation and hypotonic stress tests is inferior to that of fresh platelets.

Glycerol is a non-toxic cryopreservative but its use demands rapid freezing rates of 30°C per minute and the resulting platelet concentrate must be stored in liquid nitrogen. Glycerol stored platelets show variable recovery and survival rates in general slightly inferior to those of DMSO-cryopreserved platelets.

The use of macromolecules such as hydroxyethyl starch (HES), and ficoll as cryopreservatives as well as the addition of prostacyclin analogues to improve function after cryopreservation are under investigation.

Indications for platelet transfusion

In the introduction to this section the importance of platelets in maintaining primary haemostasis was outlined. The normal platelet count is $150-400 \times 10^9/l$ and the marrow produces around 35×10^9 platelets daily, with a lifespan of 9–10 days. In conditions of platelet consumption the marrow is able to increase its output sixfold. However, even if decompensation or marrow failure occurs, in otherwise uncomplicated thrombocytopenia the condition remains asymptomatic until the count drops to below $80 \times 10^9/l$. At this level trauma, surgery or biopsy procedures will result in excessive blood loss. As the level drops further to around $50 \times 10^9/l$ minimal trauma may produce superficial bruising and bleeding from mucosal surfaces. Platelet levels below $10–20 \times 10^9/l$ are associated with the risk of severe spontaneous haemorrhage.

From this it can be seen that any patient requiring elective surgery or biopsy should have a platelet count of $80 \times 10^9/l$ or above. Apart from this patients with platelet counts over $50 \times 10^9/l$ need only careful clinical observation. Patients with platelet counts of under $20 \times 10^9/l$ may need prophylactic platelet infusion to prevent life-threatening spontaneous haemorrhage. However, these are only general guidelines. Some individuals tolerate platelet levels of $10 \times 10^9/l$ without serious bleeding, some with levels of $50 \times 10^9/l$ suffer severe haemorrhage. An acute fall in the platelet count seems more dangerous than a chronically low platelet level. Infection appears to interfere with haemostasis, making haemorrhage at a given platelet count more likely. Dilution of an already low platelet count by blood or electrolyte transfusion may precipitate bleeding in a previously stable thrombocytopenic patient. Therefore constant clinical evaluation is needed in deciding whether platelet support is indicated. As a rule patients with cutaneous petechiae and purpura only do not require support, but those with retinal, gastrointestinal or genitourinary haemorrhage or excessive oro-nasal bleeding do.

The cause of thrombocytopenia must also be taken into account. In general thrombocytopenia due to failure of marrow production responds well to replacement therapy; that due to splenic sequestration or peripheral platelet destruction responds poorly. Thus patients with aplastic anaemia, the acute leukaemias, carcinomatosis or those undergoing cytoreductive therapy will be candidates for platelet support. Those with platelet destruction due to autoantibodies are best treated with high dose steroids, as transfused donor platelets will be rapidly destroyed. In these patients platelets should be reserved for life-threatening haemorrhage, for example, prior to emergency splenectomy in a bleeding patient who has failed to respond to steroids. Very large doses may need to be given.

Isoimmune platelet destruction occurs in Pl^{A1} positive neonates born to Pl^{A1} negative mothers, sensitized during this or a previous pregnancy, or by a Pl^{A1} positive transfusion. The neonate may have severe purpura and require platelet support using maternal platelets, washed to remove antibody. Pl^{A1} negative donors, if available, could also be used.

In disseminated intravascular coagulation the inappropriate activation of platelets is a major initiating factor, the resulting thrombocytopenia is best reversed by treatment of the precipitating sepsis or obstetric problem. However, it may occasionally be necessary to give platelets as well as fresh frozen plasma to secure haemostasis during management.

Thrombotic thrombocytopenia purpura, and haemolytic uraemic syndrome, also involve intravascular platelet activation and this may be due to a reduction in endothelial prostacyclin activity. Platelet infusions are contraindicated as these may aggravate this problem which may respond to repeated transfusions of fresh plasma or plasma exchange with FFP.

Splenic sequestration is rarely the cause of severe thrombocytopenia unless splenomegaly is accompanied by other factors such as bone marrow infiltration or cytotoxic therapy. In such cases higher doses of platelets than normal need to be given to correct thrombocytopenia.

In severe conditions of congenital platelet malfunction, patients with a significantly prolonged template bleeding time, i.e. > 15 minutes, severe bleeding may occur. Support with normal platelets should be reserved for situations associated with significant risk of haemorrhage such as trauma or surgery. Occasionally severe bleeding occurs postoperatively in patients who have been given aspirin and this responds to platelet transfusion.

The haemorrhagic tendency in myeloma is sometimes associated with thrombocytopenia. However, this responds badly to platelet replacement because the abnormality is probably due to interference by the circulating paraprotein with platelet–capillary wall interaction. The treatment is that of myeloma itself and reduction of any paraprotein present.

In uraemia the bleeding tendency may be associated with thrombocytopenia, but this also responds badly to platelet replacement as the primary defect is due to defective platelet function caused by the uraemic state. Any platelets given will of course be similarly affected, unless the uraemia is treated at the same time by dialysis.

Dosage and administration of platelets

Having decided that platelet support is appropriate the dosage required has to be estimated. A unit of platelet concentrate contains approximately 5×10^{10} platelets. Thus in an adult with marrow failure rather than peripheral destruction, transfusion of one unit would be expected to produce an increment of approximately $10 \times 10^9/l$ in the platelet count (assuming a blood volume of 5 litres). In practice recovery of stored platelets is less than 100% (Table 6.2) and 6 units of platelets is the standard dose for adults. From Table 6.2 it would be expected that the life span of transfused stored platelets would be around five days. However, this is rarely the case. Thrombocytopenic patients show a reduced life span even for endogenous platelets; the normal life span of nine to ten days being reduced to five days. Presumably this is due to increased utilization of any platelets present to stop bleeding due to the defect in primary haemostasis. Any transfused platelets are also consumed in this way. Patients requiring platelets often have other problems such as infection, carcinomatosis or leukaemia which increase platelet consumption, or splenomegaly causing platelet sequestration. HLA or platelet specific antibodies may develop after repeated transfusions from random donors. Therefore 6 units of platelets must be given at least daily in most situations, with careful monitoring of the patient for mucosal bleeding, and laboratory evaluation of the platelet count. If the platelet count one hour after transfusion of 6 units fails to rise by $40-50 \times 10^9/l$ sensitization is probable (particularly if the patient experiences febrile reactions during treatment). HLA matched related donors may then be necessary.

ABO and Rh compatible platelets are used whenever possible. Rh compatible donors must be selected because any contaminating D-positive red cells present may sensitize a D-negative recipient. In a woman of childbearing age this would be particularly undesirable. If absolutely unavoidable due to problems of supply in urgent situations, platelet concentrates from D-positive donors for D-negative recipients are preceded by anti-D immunoglobulin prophylaxis; an intravenous preparation is available and is preferred.

Platelet concentrates should be rapidly infused through narrow bore giving sets to minimize losses. Standard in-line transfusion filters should be used. Those designed to remove microaggregates (Pall 40 μm, Fenwal 20 μm pore-size) also remove platelets.

Hazards of platelet replacement therapy

These can be divided into two categories: infective and immunological.

Infective hazards

These are similar to those of blood transfusion in general (page 121). Related donors used to obtain HLA compatible platelets should be screened for HBsAg and syphilis.

In the UK over 50% of blood donors are likely to be cytomegalovirus-antibody (CMV) positive and are probably carrying latent virus. Platelets contaminated with leucocytes from such donors are only likely to cause serious infections in the severely immunocompromised or in neonates. In such cases, for example potential marrow transplant recipients, CMV negative blood and blood products should be used if possible if the recipient and donor are CMV antibody negative.

Bacterial contamination is rare if aseptic venepuncture and closed system sterile packs are used during preparation. However, some platelet-pheresis machines employ an 'open' procedure and donations from these must be used within 24 hours. Similarly reconstituted frozen platelets should be used within 12 hours.

Immunological problems of platelet infusions

Alloimmunization is usually due to HLA antigens, and the presence of contaminating leucocytes, which express these more strongly than platelets, is thought to increase the chance of sensitization. This results in febrile transfusion reactions and failure to achieve the expected platelet increment or therapeutic response. Once it occurs HLA compatible related donors should be sought. Alternatively in patients requiring long-term support such as potential marrow transplant recipients HLA matched donations may be used from the outset. Rhesus immunization is due to contaminating red cells and has already been discussed (page 87).

Platelet specific immunization is likely in the 2% of Pl^{A1} negative individuals if they are transfused and results in post-transfusion purpura as endogenous platelets aggregate with immune damaged donor cells. It develops five to ten days after transfusion with blood or platelets and may require treatment by plasmapheresis to remove the antibody.

As with any blood product febrile and anaphylactic reactions may occur due to sensitization to foreign proteins. They are treated by hydrocortisone and antihistamines.

Lymphocyte contamination of platelet concentrates occurs, particularly in those obtained by plateletpheresis and these large numbers of viable cells may cause graft versus host reaction in immunocompromised patients or neonates. This can be prevented by irradiation of the platelets before transfusion.

The plasma from some group O donors contains high titre anti-A or -B and the use of platelet concentrates from such donors to group A recipients has rarely caused haemolysis.

Further reading

Slichter, S J, Harker, L A (1976) Preparation and storage of platelet concentrates, I. Factors influencing the harvest of viable platelets from whole blood, *British Journal of Haematology*, **34**, 395.

II. Storage variables influencing platelet viability and function, *British Journal of Haematology*, **34**, 403.

Laboratory evaluation of platelets for transfusion (1981) Eds. Fratantoni, J C, Mishler, J M, *Vox Sanguinis*, **40**, supplement 1.

Law, P, Merryman, H (1982) Cryopreservation of platelets: current status. *Plasma Therapy*, **3**, 317.

Slichter, S J (1982) Indications for platelet transfusions. *Plasma Therapy*, **3**, 259.

Gilcher, R O (1982) Blood and apheresis products. Usage in modern transfusion therapy. *Plasma Therapy*, **3**, 27.

7 Granulocyte replacement therapy

Modern treatment of potentially curable malignant disorders such as the acute leukaemias by cytotoxic chemotherapy and bone marrow transplantation causes severe neutropenia. Since platelet therapy has reduced mortality related to haemorrhage, infection has become the major hazard to such patients. Measures to reduce infection-related mortality include broad spectrum bactericidal antibiotics, gut decontamination and patient isolation. However, direct replacement of granulocytes is possible and may be necessary when severe infection in neutropenic patients fails to respond to other forms of treatment.

Granulocyte collection

The daily turnover of granulocytes in the healthy adult is 1×10^{11} cells, and in septicaemia this is probably increased eightfold. Therefore useful numbers for the septicaemic, neutropenic patient cannot be procured from standard blood donations. Because granulocytes express HLA antigens strongly they are even more likely to sensitize non-compatible recipients than platelets, and hence ideally donors should be HLA compatible relatives, but if they are potential bone marrow donors they should not be used. Neutrophils also carry neutrophil specific antigens (page 27). Neutrophils are usually collected from single donors by leukapheresis. This can be done by passing anticoagulated donor blood through a cell separator (page 180), which involves continuous or intermittent centrifugation to separate cells from plasma according to their relative density. Large numbers of platelets are included in the concentrate, and the yield is sub-optimal. To improve the separation it is now standard practice to give the donor steroids before leukapheresis (e.g. 60 mg prednisolone 12 hours before donation), and to add a red cell sedimenting agent such as hydroxyethyl starch with the anticoagulant. With such methods around $1-2 \times 10^{10}$ granulocytes can be collected in a session lasting two to four hours.

Filtration leukapheresis utilizes the capacity of granulocytes to adhere to fibres. Anticoagulated donor blood is passed over nylon wool filters. The adherent granulocytes are then eluted using ACD plasma and concentrated by centrifugation. The yield from filtration leukapheresis is higher and purer than that from centrifugation, and the process is cheaper, but such granulocytes are functionally inferior and more liable to cause reactions. A serious drawback to the technique is that the donors suffer unpleasant side effects due to complement activation. For these reasons this technique is no longer used.

Patients with newly diagnosed chronic granulocytic leukaemia can be used as donors producing high yields of granulocytes by leukapheresis, or even by simple sedimentation of venesected blood.

Storage of granulocytes

Granulocytes stored at $4°C$ in CPD plasma retain nearly normal phagocytic, chemotactic and bactericidal activity for 24 hours with rapid loss of function during the next 24 hours. They are therefore usually transfused within 12 hours of collection. Cryopreservation of granulocytes has not been successful and there are no methods available for long-term storage of these cells.

Quality of granulocyte preparations

As with other blood products the ideal granulocyte concentrate will show unimpaired viability and function *in vivo* and *in vitro* when compared with freshly drawn cells. It should also be shown to be of therapeutic benefit in the infected neutropenic patient. If autologous granulocytes obtained by simple phlebotomy are radioisotopically labelled and reinfused into normal subjects recovery is only 50%, half the cells joining the 'marginal pool' of granulocytes. The survival in the circulation is only six hours in normal subjects and is even less in patients with septic foci to which granulocytes actively migrate. Any HLA incompatibility between donor and recipient would also shorten survival further once sensitization had occurred.

Studies with granulocyte concentrates obtained by centrifugation show normal post-transfusion recovery rates and survival times. *In vitro* studies of granulocyte function such as the nitro blue tetrazolium reduction test, assays of oxygen consumption and chemotaxis show that neutrophils retain normal function. Granulocytes from donors with chronic granulocytic leukaemia (CGL) show defective phagocytosis, but as they are available in high numbers this seems not to prevent therapeutic effect.

Indications for and use of granulocyte transfusions

Because therapeutically useful numbers of granulocytes can only be obtained by expensive time-consuming procedures that are not without hazard to the donor, indications for their use must be carefully assessed. Eighty per cent of patients with sepsis associated with neutropenia will respond to modern wide spectrum bactericidal antibiotic combinations. Therefore, granulocyte replacement therapy is reserved for those patients with severe sepsis, associated with potentially reversible neutropenia of less than 0.5×10^9/l, which has failed to respond to at least 48 hours of appropriate antibiotic therapy.

In controlled trials it has been shown that only cases with documented bacterial sepsis benefit from granulocyte replacement, and that therapy with at least 2×10^{10} granulocytes daily must continue for a minimum of four days, or until the fever subsides. The use of suboptimal amounts of granulocytes is a waste of effort. Granulocytes are not used prophylactically even in severely neutropenic patients as this has not been shown to improve survival, and exposes the patients to the hazards of granulocyte transfusion. In BMT recipients CMV infection has been found to correlate with the number of granulocyte transfusions received.

Selection of donors

Donors should be ABO and rhesus group matched because of red cell contamination of most granulocyte preparations. They should also be HLA compatible or ideally HLA identical with the recipient. If such donors are not available, CGL or random granulocytes may be used until sensitization develops. If it is likely that the recipient has been sensitized to leucocytes by previous transfusion of blood or blood products, leukoagglutinins for donor granulocytes should be excluded. HLA incompatibility may be demonstrated by the presence of lymphocytotoxic antibodies to donor lymphocytes. Only donors negative in both tests should be chosen.

Hazards of granulocyte transfusion

The hazards associated with granulocyte transfusion are those due to immune reactions, those associated with transmission of infection and those peculiar to the use of chronic granulocytic leukaemia (CGL) granulocytes.

Immunologically mediated hazards

Alloimmunization to neutrophil specific or HLA antibodies is risked if random donors are used. As discussed above ideally HLA identical, ABO and Rh compatible donors should be selected. If HLA compatible donors are not available and the patient has previously received blood products or has evidence of white cell sensitivity, his serum should be cross-matched against the potential donor's granulocytes and lymphocytes to detect leukoagglutinins and lymphocytotoxic antibodies respectively.

Transfusion of granulocytes to a sensitized recipient will be ineffective. More importantly it may result in febrile reactions or anaphylactic shock, and is one cause of pulmonary infiltration associated with granulocyte therapy.

Diffuse pulmonary infiltration following granulocyte therapy is more likely if there is pre-existing pulmonary pathology. It may be caused by pulmonary accumulation of cells aggregated by host leukoagglutinins. Another mechanism may be damage to pulmonary endothelium as granulocytes are activated by circulating bacterial endotoxins, resulting in release of granulocyte enzymes and complement activation. The occurrence of pulmonary infiltrates may be aggravated by the concomitant administration of amphotericin B. Pulmonary infiltration by leucocyte microaggregates forming *in vitro* should be prevented by the use of in-line filters.

Patients who develop respiratory distress during granulocyte therapy should have the transfusion terminated and receive 100 mg to 500 mg hydrocortisone intravenously. Hydrocortisone and chlorpheniramine are also used to treat febrile and anaphylactic reactions.

Graft versus host disease

This problem is due to immune activity of donor lymphocytes against recipient antigens in the immunocompromised. Patients at risk include allograft recipients and premature neonates. T lymphocyte contamination is usual in donations prepared by centrifugation leukapheresis.

Graft versus host disease can be prevented if blood and blood products for severely immunosuppressed individuals are irradiated to 15Gy, preventing lymphocyte replication on subsequent transfusion.

Transmission of infection

As with any other blood product hepatitis, syphilis and bacterial infection may be transmitted by granulocytes. Donors should be negative for HBsAg and serological tests for syphilis.

A particular hazard for the immunocompromised patient receiving granulocytes is the risk of cytomegalovirus (CMV) infection. Over 50% of the general population in the UK have anti-CMV antibodies due to past infection and may carry latent CMV in their leucocytes. This has been responsible for severe fatal pneumonia in patients receiving granulocyte support during allogeneic marrow transplantation. For patients who are CMV negative with a negative marrow donor, CMV antibody negative white cell, platelet and red cell donors should be used if available. Specific CMV immunoglobulin is available if CMV positive donations cannot be avoided.

Hazards of CGL granulocytes

Despite defective phagocytosis, granulocytes from CGL donors are effective in neutropenic patients, presumably because they are available in high doses. However, temporary engraftment of CGL leucocytes (identified by the Philadelphia chromosome) has been reported in immunocompromised recipients. Because of this CGL cells are irradiated prior to use and are given only to patients with neoplastic conditions.

Further reading

Higby, D J, Barnett, D (1980) Granulocyte transfusion; current status, *Blood*, 55, 2–8.
McCullough, J, Weiblen, B J, Deinhard, A R (1976) In vitro function and post transfusion survival of granulocytes collected by continuous flow centrifugation by filtration leukapheresis. *Blood*, 48, 315–326
Granulocyte transfusion—an established or still an experimental therapeutic procedure? International Forum (1980). *Vox Sanguinis*, 38, 40–56.
Buckner, C D, Clift, R A (1984) Prophylaxis and treatment of infection of immuno-compromised host by granulocyte transfusion. *Clinics in Haematology*, 13, 557–572.

8 Plasma products

The need for an easily stored and readily transportable fluid for volume replacement during wartime led to the development of plasma fractionation for the production of albumin in the 1940s. In 1964 a method was developed for the separation of factor VIII activity in plasma as 'cryoprecipitate' which revolutionized the treatment of haemophilia. These advances and their developments have caused an ever increasing demand for plasma far outstripping the requirement for red cells. It is this demand for plasma that has stimulated recent changes in blood transfusion practice, such as the use of either plasma reduced blood or, more recently, 'optimal additive solutions' (page 52). If used consistently, these two methods would enable self-sufficiency of plasma supplies to be achieved in each country with the modern blood transfusion service. Table 8.1 shows the products available from plasma and Fig. 8.1 outlines a scheme of plasma fractionation.

Coagulation and other labile components

Fresh frozen plasma

This contains all the constituents of normal plasma and is the starting material for manufacture of the labile coagulation factors. To avoid the triggering of the coagulation cascade and consumption of these components, venepuncture must be clean and atraumatic. The collection pack must be constantly agitated to ensure adequate mixing with the anticoagulant, the donation should be completed within 12 minutes and any pack showing evidence of blood clotting or underfilling should be rejected. CPD anticoagulants are commonly used; CPD with its higher pH preserves factor VIII better than the previously used ACD.

The blood donation should be cooled to 4°C and transported to the laboratory—not more than four to six hours from donation. Plate-

Table 8.1   Plasma products

Coagulation factors
  Fresh frozen plasma (FFP)
  Cryoprecipitate (factor VIII + fibrinogen)
  Factor VIII concentrates
  Factor IX concentrates (PCC)
  Activated prothrombin complex concentrate (aPCC)
  Fibrinogen
  Antithrombin III (ATIII)
  C1-esterase inhibitor

Volume replacement fluids
  Plasma protein fraction (PPF), Human albumin solution 4.5%
  Human albumin fraction saline
  Salt-poor albumin, Human albumin solution 20%

Gammaglobulin
  Human normal immunoglobulin (HNI)
  Human specific immunoglobulin
      Herpes zoster
      Hepatitis B
      Tetanus
      (Rabies)
      Vaccinia
      Rubella
      Cytomegalovirus
  Anti-D (anti-Rh)

---

let-poor plasma is separated from red cells by centrifugation and extruded into a satellite pack within the closed system (Fig. 5.2). The procedure should be executed carefully to avoid platelet damage with release of procoagulants. The plasma is evenly distributed within its pack and rapidly frozen to below $-30°C$ for storage. The storage life is three to six months.

Fresh frozen plasma should contain less than $25 \times 10^9/l$ platelets and less than 1×10^{12} red cells per litre. Any donation positive on HBsAG or syphilis screening will be rejected and donations containing high titre anti-A or -B are also discarded. The amount of labile factor VIII activity recoverable is a good indicator of the quality of processing and should be around 0.8 iu VIIIC per ml. After three months at $-20°C$ it will contain about 60% of its original factor VIII activity; lower temperatures will give even better preservation. Fresh frozen plasma is available in single (200 ml) or double (400 ml) packs.

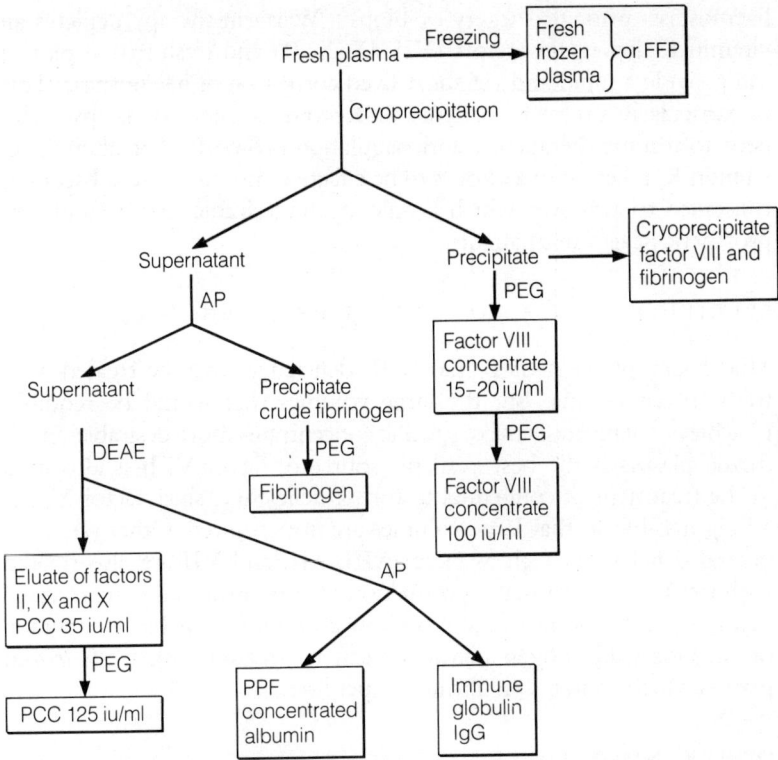

Fig. 8.1 Scheme of plasma fractionation.
   DEAE: fractionation on DEAE
   PEG: polyethylene glycol fractionation
   AP: alcohol precipitation
   ☐   available plasma products

Indications for use of fresh frozen plasma

USE IN MULTIPLE HAEMOSTATIC DEFICIENCY

Fresh frozen plasma is particularly useful in conditions requiring replacement of several coagulation factors. For example, during massive transfusion of stored blood or consumption coagulopathy (DIC), factors V, VIII and fibrinogen are particularly affected and fresh frozen plasma will replace them all. In liver disease all the coagulation factors except factor VIII may be reduced; fresh frozen plasma can restore haemostasis prior to surgery or biopsy. Warfarin therapy depletes all vitamin K dependent factors (VII, IX, X, II) and fresh frozen plasma can provide a rapid and yet short-lived correction of haemostasis. This is particularly useful in patients undergoing surgery or biopsy who need to resume therapeutic anticoagulation promptly. The alternative, vitamin K, takes up to 24 hours to be effective and can cause subsequent resistance to warfarin which would be undesirable, for example, in prosthetic heart valve patients.

SPECIFIC COAGULATION FACTOR DEFICIENCIES

Mild haemophilia A or B (factor IX deficiency) may be treated with fresh frozen plasma, but the large volumes that would be required to achieve haemostasis make specific concentrates more desirable. Fresh frozen plasma is the best available source of factor V. It is also used in the treatment of congenital factor XI deficiency, since factor XI has a long half-life so that large volumes are not required. Other rare congenital deficiencies such as factor XIII, XII, and VII are also treated with fresh frozen plasma as production of concentrates is commercially unattractive, but some of these are now becoming available. Congenital or secondary fibrinogen deficiency can be treated with fresh frozen plasma which contains 3 g fibrinogen per litre.

OTHER INDICATIONS

Fresh frozen plasma contains antithrombin III, protein C and protein S activity and is useful for the treatment of deficiency of these factors.

C_1 esterase inhibitor deficiency is an autosomal dominantly inherited abnormality causing episodes of angio-oedema. Since fresh frozen plasma contains C_1 esterase inhibitor it can be used to terminate attacks.

Use of fresh frozen plasma in clinical practice

Fresh frozen plasma should be ABO compatible with the recipient so that any group A or B haemolysins in the donation do no harm. Rhesus (Rh D) compatibility is especially important for Rh negative females, who might otherwise be immunized by red cells contaminating an Rh positive donation. The fresh frozen plasma should be thawed at 37°C, and given immediately, as deterioration of coagulation factor activity is rapid at room temperature. It should be infused as quickly as possible.

The volume required and frequency of treatment depend on the particular deficiency being treated (Table 8.2). The factor's immediate post-transfusion recovery and the level required for haemostasis must be taken into account when determining the dose, and its half-life should determine the frequency of transfusion. The activity of any factor in normal plasma is defined as 1 unit per millilitre. For example, a patient with a minor bleed due to haemophilia A, would need 10–15 ml/kg fresh frozen plasma (i.e. around 800 ml in the average adult). Because factor VIII activity is 0.8 units/ml this would raise the VIII level to 15–20% of normal, sufficient to control a minor bleed. The infusion would need to be repeated 12-hourly. The disadvantage of fresh frozen

Table 8.2 Some in-vivo properties of various clotting factors

Factor	Deficiency state	Plasma concentration required for haemostasis (% normal)	Half-life of transfused factor	Recovery in blood (as % transfused dose)
Fibrinogen	Afibrinogenaemia Defibrination syndrome	10–25	4–6 days	50
Prothrombin	Prothrombin deficiency Coumarin anti-coagulant therapy Liver disease	40	3 days	40–80
V	Factor V deficiency	10–15	12 hours	?80
VII	Factor VII deficiency Coumarin anti-coagulant therapy Liver disease	5–10	4–6 hours	70–80
VIII	Haemophilia Von Willebrand's disease	10–40	12 hours	50–80
IX	Christmas disease Coumarin anti-coagulant therapy Liver disease	10–40	18–24 hours	25–50
X	Factor X deficiency Coumarin anti-coagulant therapy Liver disease	10–15	2 days	50
XI	PTA deficiency	?30	60–80 hours	90–100
XII	Hageman defect	—	—	—
XIII	Fibrin stabilising factor deficiency	1–5	?6–10 days	?5–100

(From Rizza, C R (1976) *Clinics in Haematology*, **5**, 114)

plasma can easily be seen—the volume needed is large, and factor VIII concentrate (page 105) is preferred.

Multiple haemostatic deficiency is associated with disseminated intravascular coagulation (DIC), liver disease or warfarin treatment. Management is best guided by the results of coagulation tests: prothrombin time (PT), partial thromboplastin time (PTTK) and fibrinogen. If these are significantly abnormal, it is usual to give four packs (800 ml) of FFP to adults, but in some cases up to 1800 ml may be required to achieve haemostasis.

Following transfusion of more than 10 units of stored blood to an adult, coagulation defects may develop. Fresh frozen plasma replacement should be guided by the results of PT and PTTK tests, though some clinicians give one pack fresh frozen plasma, for every 4 units stored blood, empirically.

Hazards of the use of fresh frozen plasma

IMMUNOLOGICAL

Sensitization to plasma proteins, red cell and leucocyte antigens present in the donation may cause fever, rigors or pulmonary infiltrates. Treatment with hydrocortisone and antihistamine may be necessary. In the case of rhesus negative recipients, contaminating D-positive cells may induce anti-D formation.

VOLUME OVERLOAD

This is a hazard in the elderly and severely ill, because large volumes are often required for haemostasis and intravenous frusemide 20–40 mg is used to minimize its occurrence.

TRANSMISSION OF INFECTION

Because of screening for HBsAg and the small number of donors involved in each episode of treatment, hepatitis B and AIDS are unlikely to follow the use of fresh frozen plasma.

Production of coagulation factor concentrates

Fresh frozen plasma is the starting material for the production of all specific coagulation factor concentrates. Factor VIIIC and IX deficiencies (haemophilia A and B respectively) are the most common disorders requiring specific therapy. The demand for concentrates of factor VIII is particularly high. Isolated congenital or acquired deficiency of the other coagulation factors is rare and, if they arise, they can usually be treated satisfactorily with fresh frozen plasma.

Plasma fractionation

Plasma fractionation to produce factor VIII and IX concentrates involves a series of physicochemical manipulations which allow the isolation and purification of the desired material (Fig. 8.1).

Almost all procedures for concentration of factor VIII begin with cryoprecipitation. Fresh frozen plasma is allowed to thaw slowly; at 4°C a precipitate forms which contains over 50% of the original factor VIII activity and substantial amounts of fibrinogen. The cryoprecipitation procedure is simple and is performed at most blood transfusion centres. The supernatant plasma is removed by extrusion from each pack of FFP to a satellite pack within the closed system. The 'cryo' can be stored at −30°C for up to six months.

Large scale and commercial processes for plasma fractionation also commonly employ cryoprecipitation as their first step. Donations of plasma, often obtained by plasmapheresis, are pooled into large batches for processing. The factor VIII- and fibrinogen-containing precipitate is subjected to further procedures such as alcohol precipitation to remove fibrinogen. In general the greater the purity and concentration of factor VIII achieved in the final product the greater the losses incurred during manufacture, so that the overall yield from the starting plasma is reduced. Attempts to increase factor VIII levels in donors by administration of DDAVP (vasopressin) are being evaluated. Depending on their complexity, commercial processes result in factor VIII-containing products of intermediate or high purity (Table 8.3 and Fig. 8.1). The proteins found in various factor VIII preparations are given in Table 8.4. It can be seen that all preparations consist mainly of proteins other than factor VIII and 'high purity' concentrate would be better labelled 'high activity' concentrate.

The supernatant left after cryoprecipitation is used for the production of factor IX-containing concentrates. The 'prothrombin complex' of factors VII, IX, X and II (prothrombin) can be absorbed on to substances such as aluminium hydroxide and subsequently eluted and purified. Factor IX concentrates are therefore often referred to as prothrombin complex concentrates or PCC. Most manufacturers add

Table 8.3   Available factor VIII-containing products

Product	Factor VIII concentration (iu/ml)	K or R factor	storage (°C)	Notes
Fresh frozen plasma (FFP)	0.6	2	−30	Volumes needed very large
Cryoprecipitate	6–12	1.7	−30	Small pool
Intermediate purity concentrate	11–15	1.7	4	Large pool
High purity concentrate	20–30	1.7	4	Large pool
Heat-treated concentrate	15–20	1.7	4	Large pool*

* For HTLV-III negative patients, expensive

Table 8.4   Protein composition of factor VIII preparations

Preparation	(% of total proteins)				
	Fibrinogen	Fibronectin	IgG	IgM	Albumin
Cryoprecipitate	60–70	20–25	5–8	1–2	5–8
Intermediate-purity concentrate	42–50	15–35	10–12	2–5	12–25
High-purity concentrate:					
First generation	0–60	17–46	6–30	1.5–4	0.3–3.5
Second generation	<1–80	2–30	<3–30	5–15	2–40

(From McClelland and Yap, 1984)

a small amount of heparin to their product because of the tendency of PCC to cause thrombosis due to the activation of a little of factor X. Deliberately 'activated' non-heparinized PCC (activated or aPCC, FEIBA or Autoplex) is used to promote coagulation function in patients with haemophilia A who have developed factor VIIIC antibodies. It is thought that complexing of factor VIII with factor Xa makes factor VIII unavailable to any antibodies present.

The final factor VIII- or IX-containing material is filtered to remove bacteria, some viruses and fungal spores. Unfortunately hepatitis and the AIDS virus (HTLV-III) are not removed by this process. Because processing involves pooling of large numbers of donations, any contaminating virus could become widely disseminated. For this reason the inclusion of a 'heat inactivation' stage to destroy the AIDS related virus (HTLV-III) by heating to 60°C for 10 hours is now mandatory. The heat inactivation step is controlled by spiking aliquots of the preparation with HTLV-III to show that there is a 5 log kill. Preliminary evidence indicates that such treatment does not reduce the incidence of non-A, non-B hepatitis and that there is significant loss (*c*. 30%) of factor VIIIC activity.

These products contain a highly purified and concentrated source of the factor VIII or IX, and because the activity of the batch can be assayed, the activity in each vial of the freeze dried concentrates can be stated. For factor VIII most manufacturers supply vials containing 300 units of activity for reconstitution to 30 ml volume. Thus volume overload is not a risk with such preparations. Most manufacturers supply PCC as vials containing 500 units of factor IX activity to be reconstituted to 30 ml volume.

Clinical use of factor VIII

Indications for the use of factor VIII

HAEMOPHILIA A

Here the component of the factor VIII complex that is lacking is VIIIC (or procoagulant). Its deficiency is a X-linked, recessively inherited disorder. Factor VIIIC levels in severe haemophiliacs are <1%, moderate cases have levels of 1–5% and mild cases have levels >5% of normal. Female carriers have levels of around 50% but occasionally lower values are found. The international unit of factor VIII is equivalent to 1% of normal factor VIII activity (1% = 1 iu/dl or 1 iu factor VIII is the amount in 1 ml of normal plasma).

VON WILLEBRAND'S DISEASE

This autosomal, dominantly inherited disorder has many variants. In the majority of cases there is a moderate reduction of both factor VIIIC and VIII RAG/RICOF. The latter denotes that part of the factor VIII molecule which is involved in normal platelet adherence and aggregation. In most cases there is a mild coagulation defect with a prolongation of bleeding time. On administration of plasma or cryoprecipitate these patients show a secondary rise of factor VIIIC.

DDAVP is used for the treatment of von Willebrand's disease avoiding unnecessary exposure to plasma products.

DISSEMINATED INTRAVASCULAR COAGULATION

During DIC factor VIIIC is rapidly depleted and needs replacing.

Dosage and administration of factor VIII

The levels of factor VIIIC required under different clinical circumstances have been well defined (Table 8.5). Thus the dose required

Table 8.5   Level of coagulation factor required in various conditions

Condition	Factor VIII or IX required (iu/dl)	Duration of treatment (days)
Serious accidents, major surgery	>70	10–14
Haemarthroses, dental extractions, intra-abdominal bleeding	20–60	2–4
Early haemarthrosis or muscular bruising	15–30	1 dose

can easily be determined and its frequency will be dictated by the particular condition and the half-life of factor VIIIC (Table 8.2). Products available for factor VIII replacement are shown in Table 8.3.

For safe major surgery the factor VIIIC level must be over 100% of normal and it must be maintained above 70% for 48 hours postoperatively. During the first 48 hours the calculated dose required is given 8-hourly to keep the levels high. After the first 48 hours levels of 50% will suffice until secondary healing has occurred, and the calculated dose need only be given 12-hourly. Thus treatment is continued for about 14 days. Factor VIII levels must be checked pre- and post-infusion to ensure that the desired level is achieved and that factor VIII antibodies have not developed. Suture or drain removal and activities such as physiotherapy must be timed to follow a factor VIII injection. The same rules apply to treatment of accidental trauma.

Major haemarthroses, muscle haematomas and minor surgery such as dental extractions require factor VIIIC levels of 20–60%. Doses should be given 12-hourly for one to four days.

Early haemarthroses and haematomas may be treated by a single dose of factor VIIIC, to raise the level to 15–20%. Early treatment limits bleeding and impairment of function is minimized. It also uses less material. In many centres the patient is given a supply of factor VIII concentrates to keep at home for 'on demand' early therapy of these bleeds.

Mildly affected haemophiliacs (levels of 5% or more) rarely suffer spontaneous haemarthroses. This has prompted physicians to recommend prophylactic therapy to some severe haemophiliacs, and 20 units of factor VIII per kg body weight is given every 48 hours.

For most indications patients with von Willebrand's disease require less frequent infusions, and cryoprecipitate is preferred. During production of factor VIII concentrates the VIIIvWF activity and the ability to form multimers is lost, making them less useful in this disease. DDAVP can also be used in some cases.

Choice of materials available for factor VIII replacement

Cryoprecipitate is relatively cheap, safer from the hazard of hepatitis and suitable for moderately severe bleeds in haemophilia A and von Willebrand's disease. It has to be thawed, which involves a delay of 20–30 minutes before injections. Because of pack to pack variation in factor VIIIC content one should err on the generous side when calculating the dose required. Infusion should be preceded by intravenous injection of 10 mg chlorpheniramine, as reactions to this crude product are common.

The intermediate and high purity factor VIII concentrates allow an accurate dose to be given in small volume by syringe. The freeze dried product is dissolved in a sterile solution provided by the manufacturer. The procedure is rapid and convenient and these products are preferred for home therapy. The precise factor VIIIC content and high specific activity make high purity concentrates ideal for the treatment of severe bleeding episodes in patients with factor VIII antibodies.

Calculation of dose required

The administration of 1 iu of factor VIII/kg body weight will raise the level of factor VIII in the plasma by about 1.7–2 iu/dl. The rise(K) achieved varies for different factor VIII products (Table 8.3).

$$\text{dose required} = \frac{\text{rise required (iu/dl)} \times \text{wt in kg}}{K}$$

After giving factor VIII the expected rise should be compared with the actual rise achieved.

Factor VIII replacement for patients with factor VIII antibodies

Around 10% of haemophiliacs develop 'inhibitors' or immune IgG antibodies to factor VIIIC. This does not correlate with the amount of treatment or its frequency. Eighty per cent of such patients will subsequently give the classical anamnestic response when challenged with factor VIIIC treatment, and the antibody titre will rise within a few days. These 'high responders' are difficult to manage. The other 20% are low responders and do not produce a rise in antibody titre on receiving factor VIIIC.

The antibody titre is measured by its ability to neutralize factor VIIIC activity in normal plasma. One such measure of antibody strength—the Bethesda unit (Bu)—is based on assay of residual factor VIII in a mixture of test plasma and normal plasma after incubation for two hours at 37°C. A decrease in factor VIII of 50% greater than the control is defined as one Bethesda unit of antibody activity. Measurement of the Oxford unit utilizes similar principles and 1 Bethesda unit is equivalent to 2 Oxford units. Management of patients with factor VIII antibodies depends on the severity of the bleed, initial antibody level and 'responder' status.

Low responders with low levels of factor VIII antibody can safely be given factor VIII therapy without prejudicing its use in later emergencies. Thus they can be treated for even moderate bleeding episodes. High responders with moderately high levels of inhibitor (less than 50 Bu) should have factor VIII therapy reserved for severe bleeds or surgical cover, when very high doses of factor VIII will be required to netralize the antibody. As the titre rises due to the anamnestic response, activated prothrombin complex (aPCC) may be used in an attempt to 'bypass' factor VIII. For moderately severe bleeds in such cases conservative therapy such as splinting, alone or in combination with aPCC, should be used.

In those high responders with high initial inhibitor titres greater than 50 Bu, even high doses of factor VIIIC concentrate will be neutralized, and aPCC is the treatment of choice. However, only about 65% of patients respond. aPCC is used in the same way as factors VIII concentrate. It has also been used for home treatment in some cases. Most manufacturers supply aPCC with stated factor VIII 'correction units' which correlate with clinical efficacy: 50–100 units/Kg are given and can be repeated 8-hourly. Response is indirectly assessed by measurement of changes in prothrombin times and partial thromboplastin time. The beneficial effect of aPCC is thought to be due to the complexing of factor Xa with any residual factor VIIIC protecting the latter from destruction by antibody.

Porcine factor VIII has now been highly purified by treatment with polyethylene glycol and is therefore much less antigenic. This is used in patients unresponsive to aPCC. It can often be given repeatedly over a long period of time without antibody formation. It also does not cause an anamnestic response. In addition to the above measures, steroids, cyclophosphamide and plasmapheresis may be used to reduce the inhibitor activity.

Cloned factor VIIIC

In the future factor VIII will be manufactured by cells in culture, relieving the blood transfusion service of the need to collect the huge amounts of plasma used for factor VIII production at present. But even more importantly it will also remove the possibility of the transmission of viral diseases such as AIDS and hepatitis to the patients with haemophilia.

The human gene for factor VIIIC has been cloned and inserted into mammalian kidney cells in culture. These cells secrete factor VIIIC into the medium and up to 7% of the normal plasma concentration can be detected. This protein appears *in vitro* to have all the properties of factor VIIIC but does not have the carbohydrate usually found on it. Before this material can be used clinically it will have to be purified and concentrated, processes which are undoubtedly already being developed, but this may take two to five years. When 'cloned factor VIIIC' is ready for clinical trials it remains to be seen whether it is stable enough in plasma without prior attachment to factor VIII-cofactor. Perhaps in this respect luck may be on the side of the haemophiliacs in that any injected factor VIIIC will combine with their own cofactor thus forming a stable, active molecule. If this turns out to be so, it will be of less use for von Willebrand's disease in which the cofactor is primarily affected.

Factor IX concentrates (PCC)

Haemophilia B or Christmas disease is an X-linked recessive disorder resulting in reduced factor IX activity. It has similar clinical features to haemophilia A. Treatment is with factor IX concentrate (PCC). Approximately the same levels of factor IX are required for haemostasis as are given in the section discussing factor VIII replacement (Table 8.5). Recovery of factor IX after infusion of the prothrombin complex (PCC) is relatively low, but this is offset by its longer half-life of 20–24 hours. There are many products available; most contain factors II, X as well as factor IX and a variable amount of factor VII. These are freeze dried and are stable on storage and convenient to reconstitute. PCC is also used to treat patients who are bleeding due to excess antico-agulant therapy. Deliberately activated PCC, aPCC, is reserved for use in haemophiliacs with factor VIII antibodies. Antibodies against factor IX develop rarely.

Hazards of specific coagulation therapy

Infective

Infection with hepatitis B is risked with all these plasma products espe-cially those derived from large pools. Cryoprecipitate carries the least risk. The risk of transmission of AIDS probably parallels that of hepati-tis B (page 143). Seventy to eighty per cent of severe haemophiliacs who have been treated with factor VIII concentrates are anti-HTLV-III positive but clinical AIDS has occurred in only very few such patients, contrasting with the higher incidence in anti-HTLV-III positive homo-sexuals. Five to ten per cent of all haemophiliacs (A and B) are chronic HBsAg carriers, and 20–45% have permanently elevated transaminases. In the past ten years, as efforts to eliminate hepatitis B have succeeded, non-A non-B viruses have been responsible for 50–90% of episodes of clinical hepatitis in haemophiliacs. Up to 90% of haemophiliacs will have elevation of LFTs after receiving their first exposure to factor VIII concentrate, but only 5% will develop clinical hepatitis. Heat treatment at 60°C kills the AIDS virus, but has not reduced the incidence of non-A non-B hepatitis.

Immunological hazards

INHIBITORS

Injection of coagulation factors VIIIC, VIIIRag, and IX into patients who lack them congenitally inevitably involves the risk of immuniza-tion. Fortunately, antibodies to the latter two are rare in von Willebrand's disease and factor IX deficiency (Christmas disease) respectively.

ANAPHYLAXIS

As with any other foreign material, febrile reactions, anaphylaxis and pulmonary infiltrates may result from sensitization. Steroids and anti-histamines are used in their treatment and prevention.

HAEMOLYSIS

High titre anti-A and anti-B blood group isoagglutinins may be present in factor VIII products derived from large pool donations. These cause mild jaundice, falling haemoglobin, a rising reticulocyte count and positive direct antiglobulin test in group A or B patients after large doses. The patient's marrow usually compensates by increased erythro-poeisis, but occasionally group O washed red cells must be given.

CIRCULATING IMMUNE COMPLEXES

These can be detected in the blood of many haemophiliacs. These may immobilize the reticuloendotheial system, and also theoretically cause damage to renal tubules or synovial membranes, but long-term effects are uncertain.

IMMUNE DEFICIENCY

Recently low T helper/T suppressor lymphocyte ratios have been found in haemophilia A sufferers. Haemophilia A patients may also suffer hypergammaglobulinaemia and immune thrombocytopenia. These phenomena seem to correlate with the amount of treatment given and may be the effects of repeated challenge with high antigenic loads. The risk of AIDS is due to a virus, HTLV III (page 143).

THROMBOTIC HAZARDS

Factor IX-containing products whether PCC with heparin or aPCC, can cause thromboembolism and disseminated intravascular coagulation (DIC). This is due to the presence of a small amount of activated factor X. Neonates and patients with reduced liver function, who have low antithrombin III levels, seem prone to this complication and should only be given factor IX for severe bleeding episodes.

Other coagulation defects

Factors VII, X or prothrombin

Congenital deficiencies of factors II (prothrombin), VII or X occur rarely, and are treated with PCC concentrates with the dose and frequency being determined by the recovery *in vivo* and half-life of the missing factor (Table 8.2). It should be noted that some PCCs are less potent in factor VII depending on the method of preparation.

Acquired deficiencies of II, VII, X and XII are best treated by infusion of fresh frozen plasma, since these deficiencies often occur in association with hepatic impairment, and PCC may result in thromboembolism.

Fibrinogen deficiency

Congenital absence of fibrinogen and hypofibrinogenaemia are extremely rare and seldom cause severe bleeding. Fibrinogen concentrates are associated with a high risk of hepatitis B and, since fresh frozen plasma contains 3g fibrinogen per litre, it is to be preferred. Cryoprecipitate containing 500 mg fibrinogen per pack may also be used.

Factors V, XI and XII

Deficiencies of factors V, XI and XII are all rare, and treated using fresh frozen plasma. Factor XIII deficiency is best treated with cryoprecipitate which contains 60% of the factor XIII in plasma. A factor XIII concentrate is also available.

Antithrombin III (ATIII)

ATIII is an α_2-globulin. The molecule forms an irreversible 1:1 stoichometric complex with thrombin, resulting in inactivation of the thrombin. ATIII also inactivates the other serine proteases, Xa, XIa and kallikrein, in a similar manner. In the presence of heparin, inactivation of thrombin and Xa by ATIII is greatly accelerated.

Neonates have only 50% ATIII plasma levels of adults, the adult level being reached at about six months. ATIII levels in women of childbearing age and elderly men are slightly lower than at other times. There is a drop in ATIII level at the end of pregnancy and around parturition.

Congenital ATIII deficiency is an autosomal dominant disorder. The ATIII level is usually 50% of normal or less. Clinically this results in a tendency to venous thrombosis and pulmonary embolism. Thrombosis occurs from young adulthood onwards, and may occur in the absence of the usual 'triggers'—surgery, trauma and pregnancy. It has been estimated that ATIII deficiency may be as common as haemophilia A.

Acquired ATIII deficiency is found during prolonged intravenous heparin therapy, disseminated intravascular coagulation of any cause and after surgery or trauma. ATIII levels are lower in about 10% of women taking oestrogen-type contraceptives. Protein-losing states such as nephrotic syndrome and enteropathy are also associated with a low ATIII. In liver disease ATIII synthesis is reduced and therefore its level falls. L-asparaginase also reduces ATIII levels.

ATIII REPLACEMENT

ATIII is present in fresh frozen plasma but is also available as a concentrate. It is indicated for patients with known ATIII deficiency as prophylaxis against thrombosis during surgery or pregnancy. It may be used in patients with hepatic dysfunction who require surgery, and in DIC. These patients are usually given a starting dose of 50 u/kg, then 5–50 u/kg per hour, i.v. of the concentrate.

Protein C and Protein S deficiencies also give rise to hypercoagulable states which can be treated with FFP or warfarin.

C1-esterase inhibitor

C1-esterase inhibitor deficiency is a disorder with an autosomal, dominant inheritance, resulting in excessive activity of C1-esterase. This causes episodes of angioneurotic oedema. FFP is a source of C1-esterase inhibitor but has the disadvantage that it may also contain complement components C2 and C4 which are substrates for C1-esterase. C1-esterase inhibitor concentrates obtained by polyethylene glycol precipitation from plasma are likely to become available in the near future.

Albumin-containing products

Human albumin is prepared from standard plasma donations during the process of plasma fractionation (Fig. 8.1). Briefly, the plasma supernatant remaining after cryoprecipitation is subjected to further purification, albumin being precipitated out by alcohol. Depending on the methods used, products of various purity are obtained. These can all

Table 8.6   Characteristics of albumin-containing solutions

Product	Volume (ml)	Protein (m/l)	Albumin (%)	Sodium (Meq/l)	Osmolarity	Storage (°C) (years)
PPF*	400	30–50	80	140	150	4 5
						20 3
Albumin	300	40–50	98	132	150	4 5
Albumin salt-poor	100	150–250	98	28	hypo-osmolar	20 3
FDP*	reconstituted	30–50	60	180	hyper-osmolar	20 5

* PPF plasma protein fraction, FDP freeze dried plasma

be heated to 60°C for 10 hours and so are free of hepatitis B and AIDS virus. The resulting preparations are shown in Table 8.6. They are usually supplied as solutions. Salt-poor albumin is also available (Human Albumin Solution 20%).

Six hundred millilitres of plasma protein fraction (PPF) (Human Albumin Solution 4·5%) can be obtained per litre of plasma fractionated, whereas 300 ml of albumin (containing 45g) requires the fractionation of 2.25 litres of plasma. Another albumin-containing product is whole freeze-dried plasma. However, this cannot be subjected to heat treatment and is therefore more likely to carry the hepatitis virus. It also has a high sodium content (180 mmol/l) which may result in excessive water retention when infused. Freeze dried plasma is therefore seldom used.

In-vivo properties of albumin-containing solutions

Albumin is a protein of mw 65,000 produced in the liver. Infused albumin behaves similarly to endogenously synthesized albumin. Its half-life in plasma is around 20 days. Complete distribution of albumin between the intravascular and extravascular pools takes from 7–10 days. Each gram of albumin in the vascular system has the capacity to 'bind' approximately 18 ml of water. Normally albumin is not lost in the urine. It is broken down to amino acids in the same way as endogenous albumin.

Use of albumin in clinical practice

Albumin or PPF can be used as volume replacement fluids during massive haemorrhage where they provide oncotic pressure, and 'buy time' for the cross-matching of blood. Infusion of normal saline in large

Table 8.7 The rule of nines. Calculation of plasma loss to guide fluid replacement for burn injuries

	% surface burnt
Anterior trunk	18
Posterior trunk	18
Each leg, total area	18
Each arm, total area	9
Head	9
Perineum	1

Loss of plasma = 4 ml for each % of surface burned per kg body weight in first 48 hours.

Replace lost volume with crystalloids during first 24 hours, and with albumin during the next 24 hours and later.

volumes (three to four times the amount of blood lost) can achieve a similar effect, but it is less sustained and, because there is dilution of plasma proteins, the resulting fall in oncotic pressure may precipitate pulmonary oedema. Plasma substitutes can also be used (p 191). See page 57 for discussion of management of acute blood loss.

Albumin-containing solutions are also used to replace protein loss after severe burns (Table 8.7). During the first 24 hours, however, most authorities recommend the use of electrolyte solutions only, as capillary integrity is so poor that colloids are rapidly lost.

Albumin is indicated in reversible hypoproteinaemic states such as acute nephrosis, acute liver failure and hypercatabolic states occurring after extensive trauma or surgery. It should be given when the albumin level falls below 20–25 g/l and aim to raise the level to 30 g/l. The dose must be infused over 12 hours to avoid rapid fluid shifts.

Calculation of dose required:

$2(D - A) \times PV$ = Dose of albumin in grams
D = desired level of albumin in g/l
A = actual level of albumin in g/l
PV = plasma volume in litres (i.e. 0.04 × body weight in kg)

In practice each bottle of 4.5% albumin will raise the serum albumin of an average adult by 4–5 g/l.

The use of albumin in chronic hypoproteinaemic states such as cirrhosis of the liver and the nephrotic syndrome is more controversial. The oedema and ascites accompanying these conditions should be treated by diuretics such as spironolactone and dietary sodium restriction. If the patient fails to lose weight on such regimes, infusion of salt-poor albumin may increase oncotic pressure and secure a diuresis, or enable a response to previously ineffective diuretics. However, repeated infusions of albumin in such cases would be extremely expensive and were considered unjustified in recent World Health Organization report.

Albumin-containing solutions are also required during specialized procedures such as haemodialysis of diabetics with end-stage renal disease, and hypertensive anephric patients. They are also used during cardiopulmonary bypass procedures and as replacement fluid during therapeutic plasmapheresis.

Hazards of albumin solutions

Infection

If correctly heat treated for 10 hours at 60°C, albumin and PPF are free of hepatitis risk, but freeze dried plasma (FDP) carries a high risk and is therefore seldom used.

Bacterial contamination

This should be prevented by aseptic techniques and filtration procedures.

Anaphylactoid and febrile reactions

These may occur as with any plasma product.

Hypotensive reactions

If the solutions are infused rapidly, hypotensive reactions are possible and may be due to the presence of vasoactive substances, such as kallikrein, or their activators, derived from the original plasma. The presence of IgA may give a severe reaction in IgA-deficient individuals (page 136).

The gammaglobulins

Preparation of the gammaglobulins

Gammaglobulins are obtained by fractionation of the plasma obtained from standard blood donations. Such gammaglobulin preparations consist mainly of IgG and contain antibodies to the common antigens to which the population is exposed. The product is called human normal immunoglobulin or HNI. The separation process involves precipitation with ammonium sulphate. The yield is around 4 grams of immunoglobulin per litre of plasma. It contains antibodies to hepatitis A, hepatitis non-A non-B, rubella and measles in clinically useful amounts (Table 8.9, page 118). Satisfactory products must contain antibodies to least two common antigens for which standards are available, one bacterial and one viral. The fractionation process should be capable of concentrating the antibodies at least tenfold. HNI is commonly dispensed as a 10–16% solution in 750 mg vials. Thiomersal preservative and glycine stabilizer may be present. In liquid form they may be stored for up to three years at 4°C. Freeze dried preparations are stored at −25°C.

If therapeutically useful amounts of antibody to relatively rarely encountered pathogens are required, they must be obtained from persons who have recently been immunized by the particular antigen. Zoster immune globulin can be obtained from volunteer donors found to have high titres of antibody on screening. Tetanus immune globulin can be obtained after immunization of volunteers with toxoid. Anti-D for the prevention of haemolytic disease of the newborn (see page 160) can be obtained for Rh negative persons known to have high anti-D titres. Alternatively Rh negative volunteers (males or post-menopausal females) are deliberately immunized with Rh positive red cells. Some antibodies are found more commonly in certain groups, for instance, homosexuals have a high incidence of both hepatitis B and CMV (cytomegalovirus) infections and can be used as a source of these antibodies, but as they are also at high risk for carriage of the AIDS virus such plasma is not now used.

In order to obtain sufficient volumes of plasma, donors for specific antibody are subjected to plasmapheresis. The product is called specific immunoglobulin. For the commoner antigens most countries state a minimum level of antibody that must be present in such preparations. For both HNI and specific immunoglobulins, 80% of the protein should be intact, since aggregated or fragmented molecules can cause severe reactions on subsequent infusion. Because of the tendency of immunoglobulins to cause reactions the intramuscular injection route has been preferred. However, recent refinements in the preparation process have enabled products suitable for intravenous use to be made. The methods used and the characteristics of the resulting products are outlined in Table 8.8. Essentially, the preparation obtained by sim-

Table 8.8   IgG preparations for intravenous use—examples

Preparation	Characteristics of product
Cold ethanol fractionation followed by:	
Pepsin treatment	70–80% fragments; Fc region removed; short half-life; not opsonically active; no hepatitis risk
Plasmin treatment	50–60% fragments; Fc region removed; short half-life; no hepatitis risk; not opsonically active
Beta-propiolactone treatment	85% monomeric IgG; Fc region intact but altered; no hepatitis risk
Reduction by dithiothreitol and alkylation with iodoacetamide	More than 80% monomeric; Fc region intact but altered; no hepatitis risk; opsonically active
pH4 and low-dose pepsin	More than 80% monomeric; Fc region intact; no hepatitis risk; opsonically active
Chromatographic separation (various methods)	Well-preserved, intact and functional IgG; not yet proven to be free from risks of transmitting infection

(From McClelland, D B L and Yap, P L, 1984)

ple precipitation is subjected to enzymatic or chemical treatment, despite which, in some cases, important biological functions of the Fc portion, such as the opsonization of antigen, are retained.

Immunoglobulin preparations have half-lives dependent on their average molecular weights. Those produced by enzymatic degradations, containing fragmented molecules, have short half-lives of a few hours. Highly purified immunoglobulins with intact molecules have the normal half-life for gammaglobulins of around 25 days.

Clinical use of the immunoglobulins

Immunoglobulin preparations are expensive to prepare and should only be used in cases where their benefit has been proven. In general, immunoglobulins can be used to replace severe congenital deficiencies, to prevent development of viral infections in immunocompromised patients who are recent contacts of carriers of the infection or to prevent the development of severe infections such as tetanus or hepatitis B in immunologically normal individuals.

Replacement therapy

Severe congenital deficiency of immunoglobulins is rare; it results in overwhelming bacterial sepsis and death in early life unless prophylaxis is given. Disorders associated with gross reduction of all classes of immunoglobulin such as severe combined immune deficiency and X-linked agammaglobulinaemia require prophylaxis. Occasionally replacement is indicated for symptomatic transient hypogammaglobulinaemia of infancy, but low Ig levels without symptoms should never be treated *per se*.

Acquired immunoglobulin deficiency occurring during chronic lymphatic luekaemia or myeloma is often associated with susceptibility to infection, but this is best managed using antibiotics as the cost of prophylactic therapy would be prohibitive.

REGIMES FOR IGG REPLACEMENT

Formerly only intramuscular preparations were available, and with this method a loading dose of 50 mg/kg is given daily for five days and thereafter 25–50 mg/kg weekly is needed to maintain IgG levels of around 2 g/l. With intravenous preparations greater volumes can be given and high levels can be achieved rapidly. Loading doses are not necessary, and the half-life is longer, therefore 150–300 mg/kg given at three- to four-weekly intervals will maintain the desired level. The low normal range for IgG is usually chosen.

Prophylaxis for specific infections

In immunocompromised patients who are at severe risk from common viral infections, contact with known cases must be followed by prophylaxis within 48 hours. Thus children undergoing treatment (including maintenance) for acute leukaemia require prophylaxis after contact with chicken-pox/shingles and measles. Specific zoster immune globulin is required for the former.

Immune compromised individuals erroneously or accidentally immunized with live-attenuated virus vaccines may develop severe systemic illness and should receive appropriate gammaglobulin. Normal people who have been infected by rare, potentially fatal organisms should receive specific immunoglobulin. In the cases of hepatitis B and tetanus, active immunization should be performed concurrently. Table 8.9 gives the type of IgG required and dosages. A commonly used protocol for immune compromised children is given in Table 8.10.

Table 8.9 Summary of principal established prophylactic applications of human immunoglobulins

Disease	Subjects	Preparation	Dose
Hepatitis A	Contacts	HNI	0.02 ml/kg
	Travellers	HNI	0.02–0.05 ml/kg
Hepatitis B	Needle-stick or mucosal exposure victims	HBI	0.06 ml/kg repeat at one month
Hepatitis non-A, non-B	Needle-stick or mucosal exposure victims	HNI or nothing	0.06 ml/kg
Rubella	Susceptible women exposed in pregnancy (if termination excluded)	Rubella Ig	10–20 ml
		HNI	10–20 ml
Varicella zoster	Immunosuppressed contacts	ZIG or	12–25 units/kg
	Neonatal contacts	VZIG	Adult dose 5–15 ml, depending on potency
Measles	Immunosuppressed contacts	HNI	0.5 ml/kg
	Infants exposed to cases		0.25 ml/kg
Rabies	Subjects exposed to rabid animals	Rabies Ig	20 iu/kg
Tetanus	High-risk injuries in non-immune subjects	TIG	250 iu
	Treatment	TIG	5,000–10,000 iu

HNI = Human normal immunoglobulin
(From McClelland, D B L and Yap, P L, 1984)

Table 8.10   Immunoglobulin replacement regimes for hypogammaglobulinaemia

Method	Dose	Comments
Intramuscular IgG	25–50 mg/kg weekly (loading dose 50 mg/kg daily for five days)	Pain at injection site; maximum dose limited
Fresh frozen plasma	10–15 ml/kg three-weekly	Hepatitis risk (reduced by limiting range of donors). Reactions to FFP. Hospital attendance needed
Subcutaneous administration of standard IgG using infusion pump	Infusions up to 300 mg/h can be given frequently, so high doses possible and doses can be adjusted to achieve desired IgG level	Home treatment (self-administered) is possible. Patients need some training. Some patients dislike use of pump
Intravenous infusion of IgG preparation formulated for this route	150–500 mg/kg 3–4-weekly doses can be adjusted to achieve desired IgG level	High cost and needs hospital attendance

(From McClelland, D B L and Yap, P L, 1984)

Other uses of immunoglobulins

Anti-D immunoglobulin is used to prevent rhesus immunization in Rh negative females (page 160).

High doses, 0.4 g/kg by slow (1–2 hours) i.v. infusion on five consecutive days of intravenous, non-specific gammaglobulin are useful in the treatment of autoimmune thrombocytopenia (ITP), neutropenia, autoimmune haemolytic anaemia and other specific autoimmune haematological diseases. In post-transfusional purpura i.v. IgG has also caused rapid cessation of bleeding. The mechanism by which this treatment works is uncertain.

Other sources of immunoglobuin

It is now possible to produce monoclonal antibodies by hybridization of the single cell secreting the desired immunoglobulin with mouse myeloma cell lines. A well defined standardized product can be made and, provided it has the desired properties *in vivo* such as opsonization of bacteria and binding to macrophages, it may have therapeutic potential. However, the mouse protein is itself antigenic and any effect would be short-lived. Human B cells can be immortalized using Epstein-Barr virus, and clones producing the desired immunoglobulin can be expanded. This method may yield specific human immunoglobulin useful for *in-vivo* treatment in the future.

Side effects of immunoglobulin therapy

With intramuscular preparations pain and swelling occur at the injection site.

Systemic reactions are common in patients with congenital immunoglobulin deficiency, as the product is antigenic. They are also common in the relatively high number of 'normal' individuals who lack IgA because IgG preparations are often contaminated with small quantities of IgA. Systemic reactions can be immediate and severe, with anaphylactic shock, or delayed when milder symptoms such as urticaria, arthralgia and pyrexia are encountered. It is thought that reactions may be in part due to the presence of immunoglobulin aggregates which can fix complement, and of vasoactive contaminants such as kallikrein. Reaction can be prevented and treated with steroids and antihistamines.

These products may transmit HTLV-III as they cannot be sufficiently heat-treated.

Further reading

Watt, J G (1976) Plasma Fractionation. *Clinics in Haematology*, 5, 95–112.

Johnson, A J, Mathews, R W, Fulton, A J (1984) Approaches to plasma fractionation for improved recovery and the development of potentially useful clinical factors. *Clinics in Haematology*, 13, 3–15.

Rizza, C R (1984) The management of patients with coagulation factor deficiency. In: *Human Blood Coagulation, Haemostasis and Thrombosis* Ed. Biggs, R. Blackwell Scientific Publications, Oxford.

McClelland, D B L, Peng, Lee Yap (1984) Clinical use of immunoglobulins. *Clinics in Haematology*, 13, 39–74.

WHO Bulletin (1981) Indications and contraindications for the use of albumin solutions. In: *The Collection Fractionation Quality Control and Uses of Blood and Blood Products*. WHO, Geneva, pp. 26–35.

Brozovic, M (1981) *Acquired Disorders of Blood Coagulation in Haemostasis and Thrombosis* (Eds. Bloom, A L, Thomas, D P) pp. 411–438, Churchill Livingstone, Edinburgh.

Jones, P (1980) *Haemophilia Home Therapy*. Pitman Publishing, London.

Brownlee, G G, Rizza, C (1984) Clotting factor VIII cloned. *Nature*, 312, 307.

WHO (1982) Appropriate uses of human immunoglobulin in clinical practice. *Memorandum from an IUUS/WHO meeting in Bulletin of the World Health Organization*, 60, 43.

9 Hazards of blood transfusion

In the previous chapters the useful effects of blood transfusion and the use of blood products have been discussed. However, every time blood is used there is a finite risk of significant hazard. It is extremely important to understand the nature of such reactions so as to minimize their incidence. Blood and blood products should not be used without a clear indication to justify any risks involved in the transfusion. There are three main categories of transfusion hazard:

1 Haemolytic transfusion reactions and sensitization to blood group antigens.
2 Pyrexial, non-infective reactions.
3 Transmission of infection.

The most important of these are haemolytic transfusion reactions because these cause 70% of transfusion related deaths, the remaining fatalities being caused by infection.

Haemolytic transfusion reactions

Clinical manifestations

Haemolytic transfusion reactions vary according to whether red cell destruction is predominantly intra- or extravascular. This in turn depends on the type of antibody involved, IgG or IgM, and the efficiency of complement fixation and activation on combination with the specific red cell antigen (page 126).

If destruction is predominantly intravascular as in ABO incompatible transfusions, an immediate severe reaction occurs. This consists of severe back pain, dyspnoea, vomiting and diarrhoea, circulatory collapse and hypotension. There may be oozing from wounds and mucosal surfaces due to low platelets, etc. caused by disseminated intravascular coagulation (DIC). Later there is renal shut-down. Renal failure results from DIC and complement-mediated damage. Hypotension will increase damage to the kidney. Finally jaundice develops. In the conscious patient the symptoms are often clear and dramatic, but in the unconscious the signs are easy to miss. Here unexplained hypotension and oozing from surgical wounds may be the only signs. Usually a transfusion of about 100 ml or more has been given before symptoms appear.

With predominantly extravascular destruction, usually due to IgG antibodies, the cells of the reticuloendothelial system ingest sensitized cells and sudden massive release of haemoglobin and red cell stroma into the circulation is less likely. Therefore the reaction is less severe, with chills and later jaundice.

The transfusion reactions described above occur when the recipient has IgM or IgG antibodies against the transfused red cells in the plasma prior to transfusion. The cross-match procedure (page 215) is designed to detect such antibodies. In most circumstances when reactions occur this is due not to failure of the cross-match procedure, but to the mislabelling of samples or misidentification of patients.

Delayed transfusion reactions

These occasionally occur in patients in whom *no* antibody could be detected or a weak antibody has been missed. Sensitization occurs either during the transfusion itself, or due to previous transfusion or pregnancy producing undetectable antibody levels. In these cases the antibody is almost always IgG and its level begins to rise after the transfusion. The rising level of antibody leads to extravascular haemolysis a few days after transfusion with unexplained jaundice and anaemia. Occasionally fever and haemoglobinuria may occur.

Diagnosis and management

1 On suspicion of a haemolytic reaction stop the transfusion of blood and continue with saline or plasma as necessary. Avoid artificial plasma expanders as these may cause rouleaux formation and hinder subsequent investigations.
2 Check the patient and blood pack identification.
3 Take the following samples from the patient:

   (i) 4 ml EDTA for haemoglobin and platelet count,
   (ii) 10 ml heparinized; this can be centrifuged and inspected for

visible plasma haemoglobin and used for the estimation of plasma bilirubin, urea, electrolytes, haptoglobin, methaemalbumin and haemoglobin,

(iii) 5 ml citrated for a coagulation screen, PTTK, PT, TT and fibrinogen,

(iv) 2 ml FDP sample for fibrin degradation products,

(v) 10 ml clotted for direct antiglobulin test (Coombs'), other antibody investigations, blood group checking and cross-matching more blood if necessary.

4 Return all blood packs and infusion sets to the laboratory for the investigation of the donor blood group, the presence of high titre donor plasma haemolysin etc.

5 Save the next specimen of urine passed to test for haemoglobin and for microscopy.

Results of the above tests should confirm the presence of haemolysis, and identify whether this is due to a 'missed' incompatibility or a clerical error. In either case the direct antiglobulin test on the post-transfusion specimen may show a 'mixed field' type of positivity, donor red cells coated by antibody being agglutinated, while the patient's own cells are unagglutinated. If lysis of donor cells has been extremely rapid, the direct antiglobulin test will be negative and does not exclude a transfusion reaction.

Comparison of blood groups of the pre-transfusion and post-transfusion 'patient' specimens and donor units may show sample or pack identification errors. The commonest cause of haemolytic transfusion reactions is mislabelling of the patient's sample.

The tests will also diagnose the presence of DIC which is thought to be due to the activation of complement and subsequent triggering of coagulation. The PTTK, PT and TT will be prolonged, platelets and fibrinogen reduced, and fibrin degradation products (FDPs) raised.

Investigation of less severe transfusion reactions may show that haemolytic antibodies were present in the donor plasma. Delayed transfusion reactions are confirmed by investigation of the recipient's serum. Commonly a rhesus antibody against an antigen not present on the patient's cells but found on the donor cells is detected (Table 14.2).

Treatment of haemolytic transfusion reactions

Treatment includes replacement of labile coagulation factors and fibrinogen using fresh frozen plasma (FFP) or cryoprecipitate and giving platelets. As soon as a haemolytic transfusion reaction is confirmed 80–100 mg frusemide is given i.v. to establish a diuresis and fluid replacement is instituted, guided by CVP monitoring, if indicated, to overcome hypotension. If anuria occurs and conservative management with protein and fluid restriction fails, haemodialysis will be necessary. Mild transfusion reactions usually require no treatment.

Finally it should be noted that physical damage to the donor red cells due to mishandling, e.g. heating or freezing, may result in a haemolytic reaction.

Prognosis of haemolytic transfusion reactions

Transfusion reactions due to intravascular haemolysis and complicated by DIC and renal failure carry the worst prognosis. The overall mortality of ABO incompatible transfusions is around 10%.

Eighty per cent of all haemolytic transfusion reactions are caused by clerical, rather than technical errors. It is important that samples from patients for cross-matching are correctly labelled giving all requested details such as date of birth and hospital number. Even uncommon names can occur more than once in the same hospital or ward.

The mechanisms of immune red cell destruction

Red cell bearing antigens to which specific antibodies have become fixed (sensitized red cells) can be destroyed by several mechanisms. Intravascular destruction is mediated by complement, extravascular sequestration is performed by splenic and hepatic macrophages. It has recently been recognized that certain lymphocytes (K cells) may be cytotoxic for antibody-coated red cells. Some T lymphocytes may be cytotoxic for allogeneic red cells in the absence of antibody.

Complement-mediated intravascular lysis and macrophage-mediated extravascular destruction are the best understood mechanisms. They can occur simultaneously, but in general one mechanism predominates, depending on the antibody involved and the efficiency with which it binds and activates complement.

Antibodies and red cell destruction

All immunoglobulins are based on a protein subunit of molecular weight 150,000 (Fig. 9.1). This consists of two heavy and two light

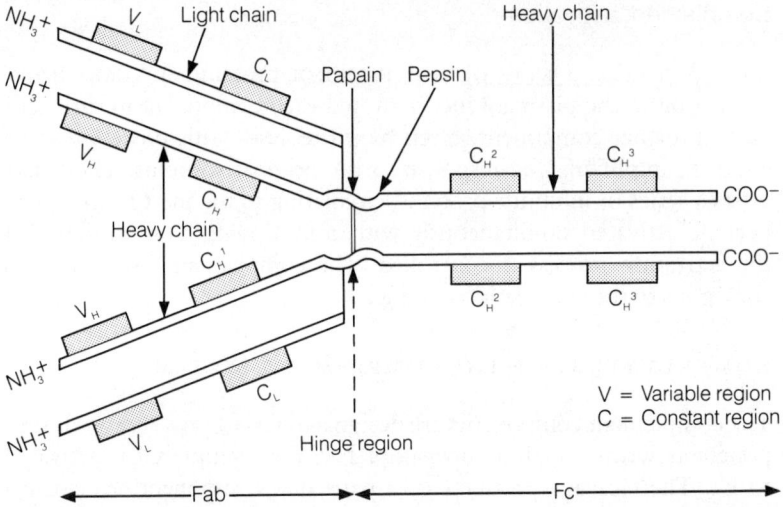

Fig. 9.1   The γ-globulin molecule.

chains joined by disulphide bonds. According to the type of their heavy chain, immunoglobulins have been divided into five classes: IgG, IgM, IgA, IgD, IgE. IgG is further divided into four subclasses: IgG1, IgG2, IgG3, IgG4.

IgG and IgM are important in red cell destruction. Because IgG reacts best at 37°C *in vitro*, and IgM at 4°C they are often referred to as 'warm' and 'cold' antibodies respectively. IgG is monomeric and IgM pentameric consisting of five of the protein subunits.

The basic immunoglobulin protein subunit can be cleaved into two portions by the enzymes pepsin and papain (Fig. 9.1). The 'Fab' portion is responsible for antigen binding, the 'Fc' portion is that part of the molecule adhering to macrophages and lymphocytes bearing the appropriate 'Fc receptor'. Macrophages have Fc receptors for IgG1 and IgG3 in large numbers, but do not have significant IgM Fc receptors. However, they do carry receptors for the third component of complement C3 the importance of which will be discussed later.

During interaction with antigen the Fc portions of antibody molecules become activated and bind the early components of complement. The Fc portions of IgG1 and IgG3 are more efficient complement fixers than IgG2 and IgG4, the last fixing complement poorly. IgM Fc is a particularly efficient fixer of complement, while IgA does not fix complement.

Complement activation

'Complement' is a series of inert precursor proteins or 'components' circulating in the plasma. Once activated each component in turn activates a further component, often by proteolysis. This process has the effect of amplifying the response to the original stimulus. There also exists a series of inhibitor proteins, circulating in the inert form, which become activated simultaneously with complement. This ensures that the activation process is controlled. The complement system is thus analogous to the coagulation cascade.

NOMENCLATURE OF THE COMPLEMENT SYSTEM

The complement components are designated C_1–C_9. An activated component is written with a superscript bar, for example C_1 is activated to $\bar{C_1}$. The cleavage products of a particular component are labelled a, b, c, d. Inactivated complement components or products are designated by a postscript i, thus inactivated C_3b is written C_3bi.

THE CLASSICAL PATHWAY OF COMPLEMENT
ACTIVATION

This pathway is shown in Fig. 9.2. Complement mediated lysis has three phases: recognition, activation and membrane attack or lysis.

Recognition
Recognition occurs when activated Fc receptors bind the early components of complement. C_1 the first component of complement comprises three subunits C_1q, C_1r, C_1s. C_1q is a collagen-like molecule, shaped like a bunch of tulips. The flower heads contain the recognition sites for the Fc portions of membrane bound immunoglobulin (Fig. 9.3).

If two of these recognition sites become fixed to adjacent Fc portions, C_1r and C_1s are sequentially activated by proteolysis. C_1q inhibitor and C_1s inhibitor control these processes.

Binding and activation of C_1q only occurs if it is attached to Fc portions of immunoglobulin at two sites. To achieve this the Fc portions must be only 100 ångstrom apart. This is easily attained by membrane bound IgM, since each molecule has five Fc portions. Monomeric IgG antibodies must be present in great density on the red cell membrane to satisfy such conditions. One thousand IgG molecules are required before one molecule of C_1q is activated. This explains why complement-

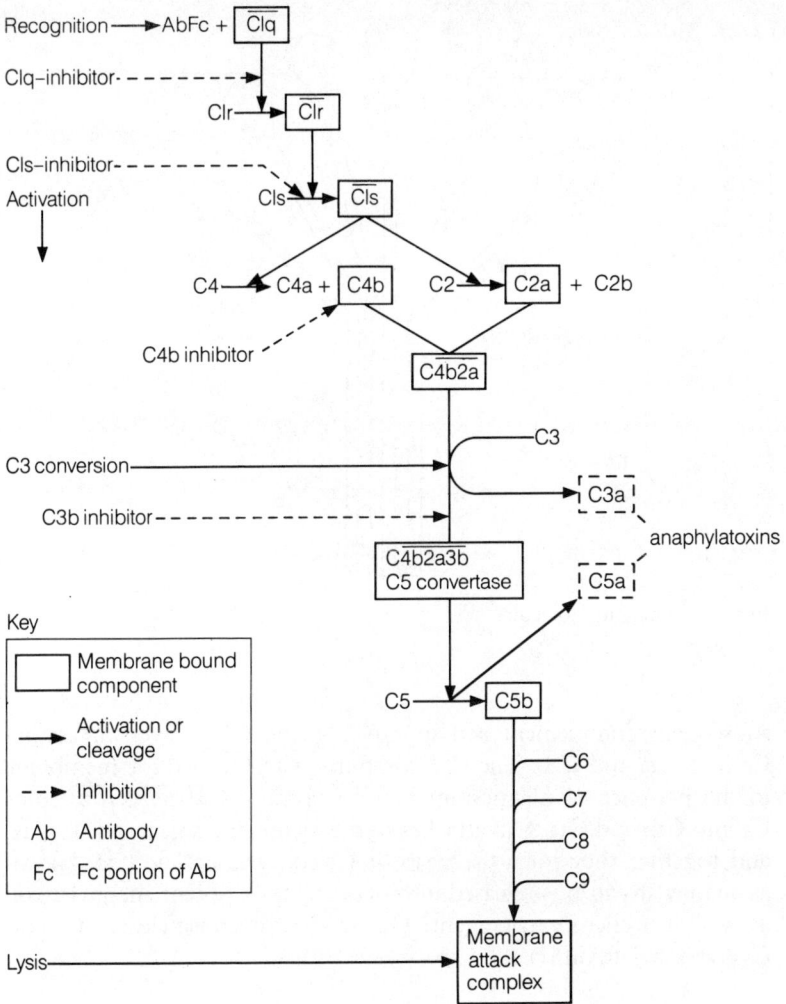

Fig. 9.2 The classical pathway of complement activation.

mediated intravascular lysis is more likely if IgM 'cold' antibodies are present.

Activation

The $C\overline{1s}$ resulting from 'recognition' acts on C4 in plasma, cleaving it into C4a and C4b. C4b attaches to the cell membrane localizing

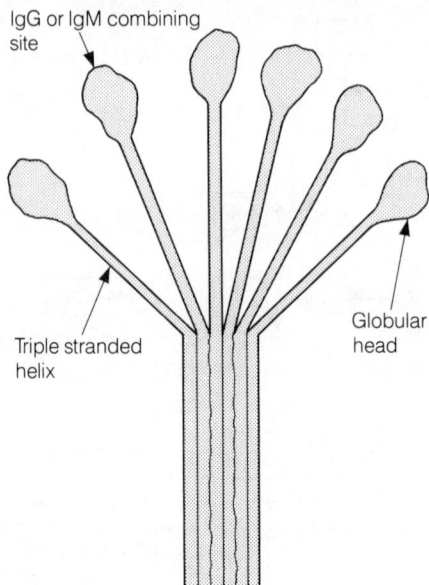

Fig. 9.3   The C1q molecule.

subsequent complement activity. In addition C$\overline{1s}$ cleaves circulating C2 into C2a and C2b. The C2a combines with C4b on the membrane in the presence of magnesium ions to produce C$\overline{4b2a}$. C$\overline{4b2a}$ splits C3 into C3b and C3a. C3b attaches to the membrane adjacent to C$\overline{4b2a}$, and together they form C$\overline{4b2a3b}$ or C5 convertase. The C3a, known as anaphylatoxin I, is released into plasma. It is a potent anaphylatoxin as well as a chemotactic agent. Finally C5 convertase cleaves C5 into C5a (anaphylatoxin II) and C5b.

Membrane lysis

C5b becomes firmly attached to the red cell membrane and complexes sequentially with C6, C7, C8 and C9. This results in a huge molecule whose hydrophobic portions insert themselves through the lipid bilayer of the red cell membrane producing a transmembrane channel lined by hydrophilic residues. This permits the flow of water and ions between the cytoplasm and the exterior, resulting in lysis.

The alternative pathway, by which C3 is activated directly, is not involved in haemolysis.

Macrophage-mediated red cell destruction

The macrophages of liver and spleen bear Fc receptors for IgG1 and IgG3, but not for IgM. They also possess receptors for C3b one of the complement products that become membrane bound during complement activation. Thus macrophages bind to red cells sensitized by IgG1, IgG3 or C3b. Of course C3b may be present on the red cells after interaction with either IgG or IgM antibody, but IgM being a more efficient complement activator more often causes completion of the reaction and lysis.

Having bound the sensitized red cell, the macrophage engulfs and destroys it. However, frequently only part of the cell is engulfed, the membrane reforming around the remaining cytoplasm, producing a spherocyte. This is a rigid cell and will be sequestered in the narrow vessels of the spleen. Spherocytes are frequently noted in the blood film in 'warm' haemolytic anaemia. In general red cells sensitized by a moderate amount of IgG are destroyed mainly in the spleen, but when a large amount of antibody is present they are destroyed in both liver and spleen. This may be because, within the narrow vessels of the spleen, there is closer contact with macrophages. Thus removal of sensitized red cells is more efficient in the spleen.

Factors determining mode of red cell destruction

From the preceding discussion it can be seen that 'cold' IgM antibodies in high titre that fix complement efficiently are likely to cause intravascular lysis. This is because many molecules of C1q can be activated resulting in the formation of numerous transmembrane channels and osmotic lysis. In some cases IgM antibodies dissociate from red cells and do not result in immediate cell lysis, leaving C3b on the membrane. In such circumstances extravascular removal by macrophages would be the major mechanism of destruction. ABO IgM antibodies usually cause intravascular lysis.

IgG antibodies, unless present in very high titre, tend to cause extravascular red cell destruction. Some IgG antibodies appear unable to fix complement, for example, antibodies to rhesus system antigens. This may be related to the number and mobility of antigens within the red cell membrane, because the distance between the Fc portions of the attached IgG must be less than 100 ångstrom for C1q binding. If too few antigen sites exist, this is unlikely to be achieved. In other cases complement activation only proceeds as far as C3b and lysis does not occur. The presence of C3b and IgG on the cell enhances macrophage uptake. In practice often both the intra- and extravascular mechanisms operate, but the predominance of one mechanism in autoimmune haemolysis can be exploited therapeutically. For example, in chronic lymphatic leukaemia with warm antibody haemolysis splenectomy will reduce haemolysis.

Autoimmune haemolytic anaemias

Autoimmune haemolytic anaemias occur due to the destruction of red cells by autoantibodies. They can be classified according to the temperature at which the antibody is most active *in vitro*, for example, warm antibodies, usually IgG most active at 37°C or cold antibodies usually IgM most active at 4°C (Table 9.1). Alternatively they are often described as primary where no associated disease can be found, or secondary when an underlying disorder is discovered. However, the longer patients are followed up the more often will the haemolysis be proved to be secondary.

Table 9.1   Autoimmune haemolytic anaemias

Underlying disorder	Common antibody specificity	Antibody class and light chain
Warm antibody mediated		
SLE	Often rhesus specific,	IgG
Chronic lymphatic leukaemia	e.g. anti-e or anti-c etc.	IgG (monoclonal)
Lymphomas		IgG (monoclonal)
Drugs (methyldopa)		IgG
Idiopathic or primary		IgG
Cold antibody mediated		
Infection		
Mycoplasma	Anti-I	IgM κ
Infectious mononucleosis	Anti-i	IgM κ
Syphilis, some viral infections	Anti-P	IgG*
Lymphomas		
Chronic cold agglutinin disease	Anti-I	IgM κ (monoclonal)
Idiopathic or primary	any	IgM

* This is a rare IgG antibody, the 'Donath Landsteiner' antibody, active at low temperatures, complement fixing causing intravascular haemolysis.

Clinical features

Autoimmune haemolytic anaemia can occur at any age, and in either sex, but its distribution is affected by any underlying disease (Table 9.1). Cold agglutinin disease, being associated with lymphoproliferative disorders, is more common in elderly males, whereas haemolysis associated with SLE is found in younger women.

Symptoms are those of anaemia, including palpitations, dyspnoea and fatigue. In addition mild jaundice occurs due to a raised, unconjugated bilirubin. The cold agglutinin diseases may be accompanied by Raynaud's phenomenon, and the intravascular haemolysis due to the Donath Landsteiner antibody causes haematuria after exposure to cold (paroxysmal cold haemoglobinuria). Moderate spenomegaly and lymphadenopathy are often present, even in idiopathic cases. Massive enlargement, however, usually indicates an underlying lymphomatous process.

Laboratory diagnosis

The haemoglobin is low, with a high reticulocyte count. The bood film shows polychromasia, and in 'warm' IgG haemolysis spherocytes are present. The diagnosis is made by the presence of a positive direct antiglobulin (direct Coombs') test (DAT) (page 209). The broad spectrum antiglobulin reagent used should be active against IgG and IgM as well as complement. Identification of the type of bound antibody is made using sera specific for IgG, IgM and IgA (rarely a cause of AIHA not covered by commercial combined reagents) and various complement components. These specific reagents are also more sensitive. The interpretation of the results is outlined in Table 9.2. In haemolysis due to 'warm' antibodies IgG with or without complement is found, while in that due to 'cold' antibodies usually only complement is found; IgM is only rarely detected. The sensitivity of the test may be increased by repeating the DAT using the antiglobulin reagents at various titres. The specificity of any antibody present on the cells and in the serum should be determined (page 215).

Treatment

Treatment is with steroids, splenectomy and transfusion. Any underlying disorder should be looked for, tests should include antinuclear factor, ESR and autoantibody screens.

Table 9.2   Interpretation of the direct antiglobulin (Coombs') test (DAT) in autoimmune haemolytic anaemias (AIHA)

Diagnosis	DAT specificity	Antibody*	Mechanism
Warm AIHA	IgG IgG + C	IgG } IgG }	(a) True autoantibody (usually within Rh, reacts with all cells except Rh-null) (b) possibly antibody to drug adsorbed to RBCs, e.g. penicillin
	C only	IgG or IgG immune complexes (IC)	(a) True autoantibody (b) Complement fixation due to innocent bystander. C fixed by IC in SLE, or drug reaction
Cold agglutinin disease	C only	IgM	Usually anti-I or anti-i
Paroxysmal cold haemoglobinuria	C only	IgG active in cold	Anti-P fixes complement in cold and dissociates at 37°C

* Antibody type confirmed in red cell eluate
C = complement

Blood transfusion in autoimmune haemolytic anaemia

There is great difficulty in obtaining compatible blood for patients with AIHA. Autoantibodies react with the cells of most donors and, more importantly, they may mask the presence of an alloantibody. Because of this, treatment of the anaemia by steroids and other immune suppressants is preferred to transfusion. However, if haemolysis is rapid and the anaemia becomes symptomatic at rest, transfusion may be unavoidable. The criteria for transfusion for other indications such as surgery or bleeding are more stringent than with other patients. Haemolysis of the transfused cells is usually no greater than that of the patient's own cells, but occasionally it may be much more severe. This may be due to relative specificity of the autoantibodies or to alloimmunization by previous blood transfusions or pregnancy.

In cold agglutinin disease special care has to be taken and the cells should be separated and washed at 37°C. For grouping and direct antiglobulin testing EDTA blood is preferred because EDTA prevents *in vitro* sensitization of the red cells by complement components.

The *direct antiglobulin test* should be done first to confirm the diagnosis. It is carried out using a polyspecific serum, but as some of the commercially available reagents do not detect IgM or IgA and may miss small amounts of IgG or C3d on the cells, a negative test should be repeated using strong monospecific sera. The recommended dilution for anti-human globulin sera is optimized for blood grouping and cross-matching and may not be optimal for detecting autoantibodies. Negative tests should be repeated using a range of dilutions of the AHG sera. If only small amounts of antibody are present on the cells, giving a negative result, these may be eluted and shown to be present by reaction with other cells.

Blood grouping

Difficulties in *ABO typing* in warm AIHA are rare. In cold agglutinin disease the tests should be carried out at 37°C. At this temperature most ABO sera react well while cold autoantibodies are usually unreactive.

In *rhesus typing* using standard 'albumin' anti-D, false positives may occur since the patient's cells may be strongly sensitized and agglutinate in albumin alone and the appropriate 'albumin only' control should always be set up. 'Saline' anti-D is preferable but commercial sera may contain small amounts of albumin leading to false positives. When using the indirect antiglobulin test for grouping, false positives may also occur. In difficult cases the antibody can be dissociated from the cells before grouping or a differential absorption technique may be used.

Elution can be done using the ZAPP reagent or by heating the cells to 50°C for a few minutes. This makes the direct antiglobulin test negative or weak, allowing an indirect antiglobulin grouping technique to be used. Control cells heterozygous for the antigen in question should also be treated in parallel to ensure the procedure does not destroy the antigen.

In the differential absorption technique equal aliquots of standard typing sera are incubated at 37°C with washed red cells known to be (1) positive, (2) negative for the antigen in question and (3) the patient's red cells. The titre of the antibody remaining in the three sera is then measured. If the patient's red cells absorbed the antibody then it is concluded that his cells carry that group.

As the genotype of patients may be important in management, all patients with AIHA should be genotyped before transfusion.

Detection of alloantibodies

WARM AIHA

Comparison of the strength of indirect antiglobulin reactions within a panel of cells relies on the probability that most of the autoantibody has been absorbed by the patient's cells and that any alloantibody is only present in the serum. Thus cells in the panel reacting with the alloantibody will give a stronger reaction than cells only reacting with the (weaker) autoantibody. Although this technique is often useful, it is not entirely reliable. This test may also reveal any relative specificities the autoantibody may have.

The patient's own cells may be used to absorb out the autoantibody leaving the alloantibody in the serum. For this the antibody on the patient's own cells is eluted (see above). These cells are then used to absorb the autoantibody from the patient's serum. This procedure is repeated several times, after which the serum is put up with a red cell panel in the usual way (Chapter 14). In order that such tests can be repeated when further transfusions are needed the patient's cells should be stored.

In the *differential absorption technique* the alloantibodies most commonly causing haemolytic transfusion reactions (ABO, Rh, Kell, Jk^a and Fy^a) are looked for. Absorption of the autoantibody is carried out with enzyme treated red cells negative for the antibody being searched for (Table 9.3). After absorption the presence of alloantibody

Table 9.3   Panel of red cells for absorption of autoantibody to search for alloantibodies, anti-Kell, anti-Jk^a and anti-Fy^a and rhesus antibodies

Genotype of cells used for absorption	Antibodies not absorbed
CDe/CDe, Kell, neg., Jk^a neg.	anti-E, anti-c, anti-K, anti-Jk^a
cDE/cDE, Kell neg., Jk^b neg.	anti-C, anti-e, anti-K, anti-Jk^b
cde/cde, Kell neg., Fy^a neg.	anti-C, D, E, anti-Kell, anti-Fy^a

is sought using the appropriate red cells. In practice only anti-Kell, anti-Jk^a and anti-Fy^a need be looked for as rhesus genotype compatible blood can be given in most cases. This method can be used in transfused patients.

After exclusion of the presence of alloantibodies, the relative specificity of the autoantibody is tested for. As the important relative specificities are often within the rhesus system, they can be identified by determining the titre to which the antibody in the serum or eluted from the patient's cells reacts with a panel of cells. The finding of such relative autoantibody specificity may make transfusion of these patients safer. The selection of blood of a patient with auto-anti-e is shown in Table 9.4.

Table 9.4   Selection of blood for patient with auto-anti-e

Patient's gentotype	Alloantibody	Blood selected
cDE/cde (R^2r)	none	cDE/cDE (R^2R^2)
cde/cde (rr)	none	cde/cde (rr)*
CDe/cde (R^1r)	none	cDE/cDE (R^2R^2)
CDe/cde	anti-e	CDe/cde (R^1r) or cde/cde (rr)

* To avoid risk of producing allo-anti-D

COLD AGGLUTININ DISEASE

One technique to exclude the presence of alloantibodies is to carry out the cross-matching techniques strictly at 37°C. On the whole this is satisfactory because any alloantibodies not detectable at 37°C are not clinically significant. Another technique is to absorb the cold agglutinin out in the cold, but this is much more difficult. The IgM cold agglutinins can also be differentially inactivated by reduction with 2-mercaptoethanol or dithiothreitol. Testing the specificity of the cold autoantibody is done using patient's serum or cell eluate against normal cord blood (i) and adult (I) group O red cells. It is recommended that the blood is transfused via a blood warming coil at 37°C.

In paroxysmal cold haemoglobinuria p or P^k cells survive better than P cells. However, as the former are only rarely available, P cells may be used, but the blood must in any case be at 37°C when it is given.

Further details of methods mentioned in this section are given in Chapter 14.

Non-infective, non-haemolytic, febrile transfusion reactions

Five to ten per cent of transfused patients have non-infective, non-haemolytic febrile transfusion reactions, but their incidence can be much higher in repeatedly transfused individuals. About 90% of all acute reactions fall into this group.

Sensitivity to white cells or platelets

The usual causes of these febrile reactions are antibodies against white cells or platelets which develop in multiply transfused patients or multiparous women. The antibodies can be directed against HLA antigens or granulocyte or platelet specific antigens.

Symptoms begin about 30 minutes after the start of the transfusion with chills and fever. Mild sensitivity reactions can be prevented with piriton 10 mg at the beginning of the transfusion and then six-hourly. Rarely, severe reactions with chest pains, hypotension, pulmonary oedema and even DIC may occur. Clinically it is difficult to distinguish these from infective or haemolytic transfusion reactions. If there is any doubt, the transfusion should be stopped; 100–200 mg of hydrocortisone i.v. may be given in addition to piriton. In sensitive patients these reactions can be prevented by using filtered blood (page 57).

Plasma associated reactions

These also occur in individuals who have been transfused repeatedly and are due to antibodies in the recipient to various plasma proteins such as IgG (anti-Gm), IgA, IgM, IgE or lipoproteins.

The Gm groups are antigenic determinants on the heavy chain of IgG and are classified according to which IgG subclass they belong, for example, Gm a is group Gm-a on IgG1. There are many different subgroups. Anti-Gm is found in pregnant or transfused individuals and in children sensitized by maternal IgG. They are also found as autoantibodies in rheumatoid arthritis.

Anti-IgA is found in IgA deficient individuals and infusion of only a small quantity of IgA into individuals lacking IgA may cause severe anaphylactic reactions with malaise, flushing, dizziness, bronchial spasm and collapse. In others in whom the anti-IgA is of limited specificity milder reactions occur.

In atopic individuals the infusion of IgE may cause attacks of asthma, urticaria, penicillin sensitivity or other appropriate response.

These reactions should be treated with antihistamines, or steroids. They can be prevented by washing of the red cells. Thus in some individuals it is necessary to use filtered, washed red cells.

Infection

Contaminated blood

Precautions to prevent significant bacterial contamination are important during collection. Because blood retains some of its bactericidal properties until immediately after collection any bacteria introduced during collection are usually killed. Such contamination occurring later is dangerous, because the blood is no longer bactericidal and is a good culture medium for bacteria. For this reason any manipulation during blood processing must take place without breaching the the pack system whenever possible. If an 'open' procedure has to be used it should be done in a sterile air environment such as cabinets designed for this purpose. Even then blood or blood products which have been subjected to an open procedure have a shelf life of only 12 hours.

Extremely rarely organisms from the pseudomonas and coli-aerogenes groups are introduced into the blood. These organisms multiply at 4°C and in only a few days many bacteria are present. The transfusion of such blood is difficult to prevent as the only sign is haemolysis, which is difficult to detect. If such blood is transfused, the reaction caused is extremely severe and almost invariably fatal. There is profound shock with DIC. The patient may vomit blood or have bloody diarrhoea. If such a reaction is supected the transfusion should be stopped immediately and supportive measures instituted. The diagnosis can be confirmed by microscopy and culture.

Transmission of disease

A number of infectious diseases can be transmitted by transfusion of blood or blood products (Table 9.5).

Hepatitis B

Before mass screening was introduced hepatitis B was the most important disease transmitted by blood transfusion. This was because a significant proportion of potential donors carry the virus involved. The disease is caused by the hepatitis B virus, HBV. The virus (Fig. 9.4) or Dane particle is 42 nm in diameter and consists of an outer coat which forms the 'surface antigen', HBsAg, originally called the 'Australia antigen'. Inside the outer coat is the core consisting of a double stranded circular DNA and a DNA polymerase. The core carries the core antigen,

Table 9.5   Diseases transmitted by blood transfusion

---

1 *Viral diseases*
   Hepatitis B
   Hepatitis A
   Non-A, non-B hepatitis
   Cytomegalovirus
   E-B virus
   Parvo virus
   Acquired immune deficiency syndrome (AIDS) HTLV III

2 *Bacterial infections*
   Syphilis
   Brucellosis
   Rickettsial infection—extremely rare

3 *Parasitic infections*
   Malaria
   Chagas' disease
   Toxoplasmosis
   Visceral leishmaniasis,
   African trypanosomiasis—extremely rare
   Microfilaria—does not transmit the disease

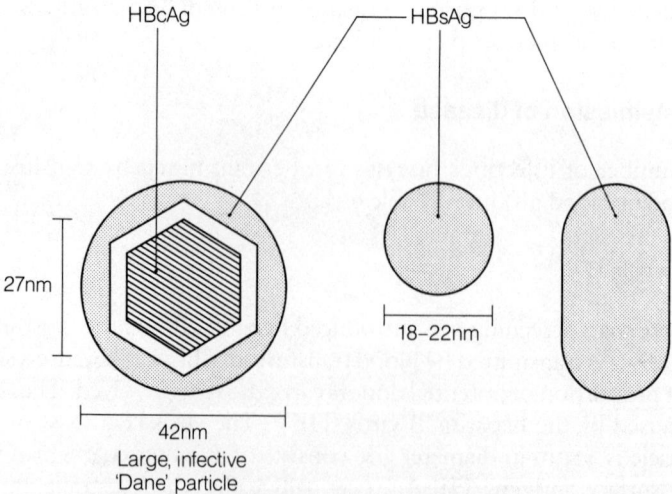

Fig. 9.4   The three types of particle associated with hepatitis B virus (HBV). (From Barbara, J A J (1983) *Microbiology in Transfusion*, Wright, Bristol)

HBcAg, and another antigen, HBeAg, probably derived from HBcAg. Two other, smaller particles can be found in the blood consisting of surface antigen, HBsAg.

The δ-agent associated with HBV is a defective virus which can only replicate in HBV infected individuals. The δ-antigen co-purifies with HBsAg. It is found in Southern Italian HBsAg carriers and in drug addicts. Infection with the δ-agent increases the severity of both acute and chronic hepatitis B.

After infection there is a two- to three-month incubation period, followed by a one- to two-week prodromal period after which the disease proper with jaundice and other symptoms of hepatitis starts. The disease usually lasts about one to two months. Most patients eventually make a complete recovery. In a small proportion severe liver failure and death may occur; others develop cirrhosis. In some the disease is entirely subclinical. The liver function tests are abnormal during the prodromal and active periods of the disease. There is no specific treatment. As the liver detoxicates many drugs, extra care has to be taken in prescribing.

During the evolution of the disease the virus particles and antigens are first found in the blood. As these disappear the corresponding antibodies take their place. The pattern of antigen appearance and antibody response is shown in Fig. 9.5. During the viraemic phase the blood

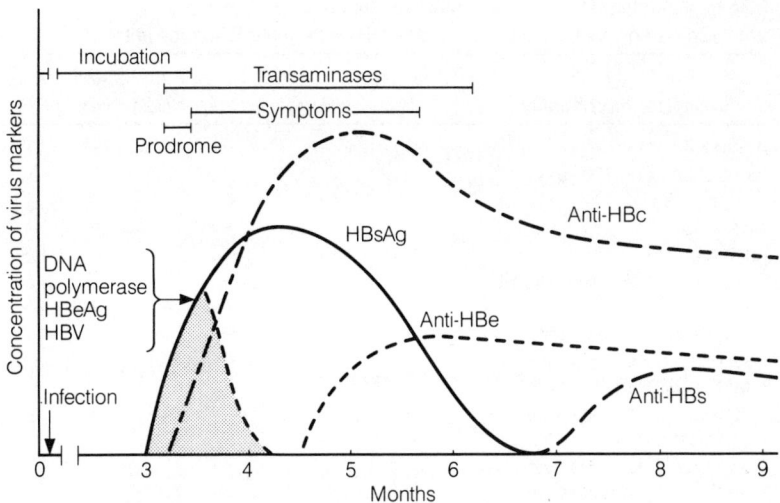

Fig. 9.5 Typical course of an acute HBV infection. (From R. Tedder, 1980, *British Journal of Hospital Medicine*, **23**, 266–279).

of the patient is infective. After the acute phase 4.6% of patients become chronic carriers of the virus capable of transmitting the infection by blood transfusion.

It is important that blood used for transfusion or for the preparation of blood products does not contain any infective virus. For this reason blood is screened for the hepatitis B surface antigen, HBsAg, using a sensitive radio-immunoassay capable of detecting 0.5 ng/ml. Any samples positive are rejected for transfusion purposes. The introduction of HBsAg screening has reduced the incidence of post-transfusion hepatitis B by over 90%. Approximately 1 in 500 of new blood donors are positive, while only 1 in 40,000 become positive between donations. Although this test is very sensitive not all infective carriers will be picked up. In these HBsAg levels are lower than the detection limit and anti-HBcAg is also present. This may occur just at the end of an attack of hepatitis B and also in a few chronic carriers. Although the presence of anti-HBcAg may suggest such a state it is not tested for routinely.

Positive donors are further investigated by measuring HBcAg, HBeAg and the corresponding antibodies. The interpretation of such results is outlined in Table 9.6. The presence of HBeAg signifies high

Table 9.6   Practical guide for the interpretation of serological markers of viral hepatitis. Anti-HA = hepatitis A antibody; HBsAg = hepatitis B surface antigen; HBeAg = hepatitis B 'e' antigen; anti-HBe = hepatitis B 'e' antibody; anti-HBc = hepatitis B core antibody; anti-HBs = hepatitis B surface antibody

Clinical interpretation	Anti IgM HA	HBsAg	HBeAg	Anti HBe	Anti HBc	Anti HBs
Acute HA	+	−	−	−	−	−
Incubation period or early acute HB	−	+	+	−	−	−
Acute HB	−	+	+	−	+	−
Fulminant HB	−	+	−	−	+	+/−
Convalescence from acute HB	−	−	−	+	+	+/−
Chronic HB	−	+	+/−	+/−	+	+/−
Persistent HB carrier state	−	+	−	+	+	−
Past infection with HB virus	−	−	−	−	+	+
Infection with HB virus without detectable (excess) HBsAg	−	−	−	−	+	−
Immunization without infection	−	−	−	−	−	+
Non A/non B hepatitis by exclusion of markers for Ha and HB	−	−	−	−	−	−

(From Barbara, J A J, 1983)

potential infectivity, because it is associated with the presence of the whole virus (Dane particle). Infectious individuals are counselled on the risks to their families and friends and vaccination is offered to these if appropriate. Individuals who are recovering from an acute infection are identified by repeat examination when HBsAg will have disappeared and the corresponding antibody will be found. The antibodies from these individuals are useful for the production of anti-HBV immune globulin, particularly after boosting with vaccine.

Laboratory personnel and others at risk from hepatitis B can be protected by vaccination, or, if inadvertent exposure to infection (for example by a 'needle-stick' accident) has occurred, by passive immunization with anti-HBV immunoglobulin. Nevertheless strict safety precautions must be adhered to. These include general laboratory precautions, cleaning of benches after blood spillage with appropriate disinfectant. When known infective specimens are handled gloves and eye protection should be worn.

POST TRANSFUSION HEPATITIS

Hepatitis following blood transfusion (PTH) should be investigated so that the type and subtype of virus infecting the patient is identified. The patient's (recipient's) serum is tested for HBsAg and, if positive, the subtype is determined. Anti-HBcAg and anti-HBcAg-IgM (the presence of IgM suggesting recent infection) are also tested for. From these results the hepatitis B status of the patient is determined (Table 9.6). Anti-HAV and anti-HAV-IgM is looked for to determine the hepatitis A status of the patient. The batch numbers and pack numbers received by the patient are used to trace the donors involved who are checked for hepatitis A or hepatitis B as indicated. For hepatitis A, anti-HAV anti-HAV-IgM is tested for. For hepatitis B, HBsAg is looked for and subtyped for comparison with that of the recipient. If the donor is negative for HBsAg, then anti-HBsAg, anti-HBcAg and anti-HBcAg-IgM are tested for to identify infective individuals negative for HBsAg (Table 9.6). Infected donors are excluded from further donations. Infected batches of blood products still available should be withdrawn.

Hepatitis A

This form of viral hepatitis is usually spread by the faeco-oral route, but is also transmitted by blood and blood products. The incubation period for hepatitis A is two to seven weeks and the disease is usually self-limiting. It is likely that blood is only infective during the prodromal period, two to three weeks before the onset of jaundice and during the early stages of the disease before antibodies have formed. Since such individuals have malaise and fever they are unlikely to donate blood and screening for hepatitis A is not necessary. If a donor develops hepatitis A, then the blood should be withdrawn or the recipient treated with human immune globulin. In 50% of the population anti-HAV-IgG can be found in the plasma.

Non-A non-B hepatitis

This form of hepatitis is now by far the most common following blood transfusion or the use of blood products and accounts for over 90% of cases. It has a variable incubation period of from two weeks to four months. Clinically it is a mild disease and subclinical infection is common. A small proportion of patients develop chronic active hepatitis. Even this complication appears to be self-limiting, resolving over a period of around two years. The disease may be due to two (or more) different viruses.

Prevention is solely by exclusion of donors with a history of hepatitis. Since the virus(es) causing this disease have not been identified, no direct screening methods are available. The possibility of using plasma transaminase levels to screen donor blood has been suggested but this has not been properly evaluated. There is some evidence that the administration of human globulin will prevent infection or modify the disease. This form of prophylaxis may be useful in individuals who receive single, very large transfusions during, for example, cardiac surgery or following road accidents. Such prophylaxis may also be useful after 'needle-stick' accidents.

Cytomegalovirus (CMV)

A high proportion (*c.* 50%) of blood donors have complement fixing antibodies to CMV and about 10% carry the virus in their white cells and can transmit the disease. The clinical features of CMV infection appear one month later with a mild febrile illness, mild splenic enlargement and atypical lymphocytes in the blood. The diagnosis is made by finding a rising titre of anti-CMV antibodies in the serum. The transmission of CMV to most individuals by transfusion is of little consequence even when massive transfusions have been given. However, in some situations CMV antibody negative individuals may be at risk.

In bone marrow transplantation CMV infection increases the severity of graft versus host disease (GVHD) and interstitial pneumonitis. Other immune suppressed individuals, particularly renal transplant recipients, are also at risk. Premature babies, whose immune systems are immature, are also at risk of severe infection. The prophylactic administration of CMV-immune globulin protects against the infection. Blood products used may also be screened for CMV infection and only CMV seronegative individuals used as donors for bone marrow transplant patients, neonates and CMV seronegative pregnant women to protect the fetus. Irradiation (15 Gy) of blood products is also used.

Acquired immune deficiency syndrome (AIDS)

This condition is a severe illness occurring mainly in homosexual males. It consists of lymph gland enlargement, general ill health, lymphopenia with reduced T-helper cells in the peripheral blood associated with either opportunistic infections or Kaposi's sarcoma. It is usually fatal within two or three years. The disease has a long incubation period of up to five years and may be preceded by a milder prodromal syndrome, the persistent generalized lymphadenopathy (PGL) syndrome.

The causative organism of the syndrome is a retrovirus, the AIDS related virus ARV or HTLV-III. This virus reacts with the T4 receptor on T-helper lymphocytes. In many individuals antibody to the virus, anti-HTLV-III, is formed, but in general these do not neutralize the virus and virus can be isolated from individuals with the antibody. It is not known whether the virus will cause AIDS in everyone infected with it, but this seems unlikely. Predisposing factors are not known, but altered immune responsiveness related to viral infection, foreign protein injection or genetic factors may be involved.

There is also an immediate reaction to infection with HTLV-III. This consists of a viral type illness with lymphadenopathy and pneumonitis occurring about two weeks after infection. After a week or so this clears up and the patient becomes positive for anti-HTLV-III. How this reaction is related to the long-term sequelae of HTLV-III infection is not known.

SPREAD OF INFECTION

Infection is spread by sexual contact and mucosal damage may be involved. It is not clear whether it is spread orally (kissing), but this is probably not a major route. The infection can also be transferred from the mother to the fetus either transplacentally or at the time of birth. It is very unlikely that the disease is spread by casual contact with infected persons living in the community. There have been no definitive reports of hospital or laboratory acquired infections except by 'needle-stick' accidents. As there are almost 10,000 patients with AIDS worldwide such infection must be distinctly unusual. In Central Africa the virus may have been present for a long time and is found equally in both sexes; it may be spread by insect vectors.

Several cases have been reported in haemophiliacs, who have received treatment with large pool factor VIII concentrates and in other patients who have had blood transfusions from HTLV-III carriers. There is, therefore, no doubt that the infection can be spread by blood or blood products. Like hepatitis B one viraemic donor can infect a whole batch of factor VIII concentrate. For this reason male homosexuals and female partners of bisexual males are now not knowingly accepted as blood donors. As the most highly at-risk population, promiscuous homosexuals, are also likely to have hepatitis B, the exclusion of HBV positive individuals from donor panels will exclude some, but not all, carriers of the AIDS virus.

The ability to isolate and grow the virus has allowed the detection of antibodies to the virus, anti-HTLV-III. Almost all patients with AIDS are positive. In the persistent lymphadenopathy syndrome about 90% are positive. In AIDS contacts and other homosexuals at risk the antibody is found in about 20–40% cases; intravenous drug abusers are about 1% positive. Thirty to forty per cent of haemophiliacs who have received large pool factor VIII concentrate are also positive and some AIDS cases have been reported. Over a thousand blood donors have been tested in London without any positive individuals being found. In future all blood donations will be screened for HTLV-III antibodies and positive donations not used.

SAFETY PRECAUTIONS

In considering the precautions to be taken by hospital staff looking after patients with AIDS or in laboratories handling infected material, the fatal nature of the disease, lack of effective treatment or prevention of infection by passive or active immunity as well as the incomplete understanding of the possible modes of spread have to be taken into account. For these reasons strict guidelines have been laid down by the Advisory Committee on Dangerous Pathogens. The patient should be nursed in isolation. It is assumed that blood, other body fluids, excreta and tissues from infected individuals are able to transmit the infection and should be handled with extreme care. The virus has been isolated from blood, saliva and semen. Disposable gloves, plastic aprons and eye protection must be worn when handling, collecting or processing such material. All specimens sent to the laboratory must be clearly marked indicating the risk of HTLV-III infection. In the laboratory specimens should be handled in a room set aside for this work with a containment level 3. All handling of material should be carried out in a microbiological safety cabinet class 1 or 3 preferably the former. Type 2, i.e. laminar airflow cabinets, are not considered suitable.

Epstein-Barr virus (EBV)

As most individuals (>95% of adults) are immune to EBV this is not of great importance in blood transfusion. In susceptible persons it can cause mild hepatitis. Individuals who have had infectious mono-nucleosis in the previous two years are not accepted as blood donors. EBV may cause lymphoma in immune suppressed individuals.

Parvo virus

Parvo virus, which causes fifth disease, specifically inhibits red cell matu-ration for a few days causing red cell aplasia. In normal individuals, because of the shortness of this effect, this is of no consequence, but in patients with haemolysis, severe anaemia may be caused, but recovery is rapid. The virus may be transmitted by blood transfusion, but this is not of clinical significance.

Brucellosis

Transmission of brucellosis is extremely uncommon. However, because the disease is chronic and difficult to treat it is recommended that people with a history of brucellosis do not donate blood.

Syphilis

This is not an important problem as the organism is only present in the blood in the early seronegative phase of the disease; it also does not survive 4°C or freezing for more than 72 hours. Finally blood which is seropositive for syphilis (TPHA) is not used for transfusion.

Malaria

The transmission of malaria by blood transfusion is an important problem which can, to some extent, be prevented.

In non-malarial areas donors who have been to an endemic zone area in the last three years should be rejected.

In endemic areas the blood may be screened using an indirect fluorescent antibody technique, but this is not always effective. Alternatively a single dose of chloroquine (600 mg) can be given 48 hours before blood donation. The recipient can be given 600 mg of chloroquine just before or after the transfusion. This should be followed by 300 mg weekly for four doses.

Storage of blood at 4°C reduces the risk of transmission to some extent, particularly of *P. malariae*. Transmission of *P. falciparum* has occurred after two weeks' storage.

Chagas' disease

This is caused by *Trypanosoma cruzi* and is only a problem where this is endemic. In Latin American 1–22% of donors may be seropositive for *T. cruzi* and about 10% of recipients of such blood become infected. Infection can be prevented by excluding seropositive donors. The addition of 125 mg crystal violet to each unit of blood kills the parasite. Storage at 4°C is only partially effective.

Toxoplasmosis

This is not a problem except in granulocyte transfusions to immune-suppressed patients and individuals with raised antibodies to *Toxoplasma* are not used as donors for this purpose.

Other hazards of blood transfusion

Citrate toxicity

This only occurs in large transfusions to patients with liver disease or those with a low plasma calcium. Treatment is with i.v. calcium p. 70.

Potassium toxicity

After blood has been stored for a few days potassium levels increase in the plasma (page 52). This is only of importance in large or exchange transfusions, for example for haemolytic disease of the newborn.

Hypothermia

If cold blood is rapidly transfused, cardiac arrhythmias may be caused. If blood is warmed prior to transfusion, the conditions should be carefully controlled as haemolysis occurs if 40°C is exceeded.

Circulatory overload

This is an important problem in patients with heart disease or with severe anaemia. These patients should be transfused very slowly with washed, packed cells; it may be necessary to give only one or two units at a time with a 24-hour gap between transfusions. Diuretics should also be used (page 67).

Transfusional iron overload

Each unit of blood contains about 250 mg of iron and in patients who are transfused regularly for anaemia iron overload occurs after one to two years when more than 20 g of iron have been given. The toxic effects of transfused iron are the same as those in haemochromatosis.

Liver damage leading to cirrhosis

Endocrine damage

  Diabetes
  Hypoparathyroidism
  Failure to grow
  Delayed puberty
  Loss of libido

Cardiac damage

  This consists of various arrhythmias as well as cardiac failure due to cardiac myopathy. It is the most common cause of death.

Skin pigmentation

Liability to infection

Prevention and treatment of these complications is by the removal of iron using parenteral desferrioxamine. When this is used in adequate doses early in the transfusion regime it will prevent iron accumulation. Moderate pathology is usually reversible. Desferrioxamine, 50 mg/kg/day, is given subcutaneously over 12 hours by a syringe pump five to six times each week. Fifty to one hundred milligrams ascorbic acid are given orally prior to the infusion to increase iron mobilization. Higher doses of desferrioxamine, up to 125 mg/kg, can be used i.v., but doses above this level cause eye and possibly CNS toxicity.

Phlebitis

This is an important complication and prevention is by using sterile precautions and careful technique.

Air embolism

These are avoidable by careful technique. If blood is to be given more rapidly than is possible by gravity, a suitable pump should be used.

Further reading

Barbara, J A J, Tedder, R S (1984) Viral infections transmitted by blood and its products. *Clinics in Haematology*, **13**, 693.
Barbara, J A J (1983) *Microbiology in Blood Transfusion*. John Wright, Bristol.
Seminars in Haematology (1981) **18**, 84–146.
Advisory Committee on Dangerous Pathogens (1984) *Acquired Immune Deficiency Syndrome (AIDS)—Interim Guidelines*. Department of Health and Social Security, London.
Gilcher, R O (1985) Transfusion related complications. *Plasma Therapy Transfusion Technol*. **6**, 3–128.

10 Transfusion in neonatal medicine

The principles of transfusion in the newborn are essentially similar to those in the adult, but great care has to be taken because of the small size of the baby, particularly if it is premature. The blood volume per kilogram of body weight is larger than that of an adult and 90 ml/kg is used for calculating the circulating blood volume and estimating the amount of blood to be given. Using this value it can be seen that in a normal, 3.5 kg newborn 30 ml of whole blood is equivalent to a unit of blood in an adult. Therefore any blood lost (or taken for clinical investigations) forms a larger proportion of the total blood volume of the baby concerned. If one tenth or more of the blood volume is taken for investigations it would need to be replaced by transfusion. It also has to be remembered that the coagulation system and the immune system are not fully developed at birth. All these factors affect premature and small-for-dates infants more than full term, normal neonates.

At birth the oxygen affinity of the blood is significantly higher than that of adults, with a P_{50} of 2.9 kp (22 mmHg) compared to 3.5 kp (26.5 mmHg) for adults. Shortly after birth the 2,3DPG level in the fetal cells rises so that the oxygen affinity becomes the same as that of adult blood. It has been suggested that transfusion of adult cells *per se* would be of value to infants, but because of the adjustment of the oxygen affinity of fetal cells this is not so. If the neonate is acidotic, this will affect the oxygen affinity of fetal and adult cells to the same extent and transfusion is of no benefit. Therefore transfusions should only be given for specific indications.

Newborn babies have a more exacting requirement than adults. Donors should be screened as for transfusion in adults (page 228) but should also be anti-CMV negative. The blood should have a near normal plasma potassium, a pH of 7.2 and a normal red cell 2,3DPG. The blood should also be plasma reduced to a haematocrit of 0.65. Because of the small volumes needed, small, multiple, CPD plastic bag collection systems are available with which suitable 'baby packs' of plasma-reduced blood can be produced. Such blood is used for up to three days for exchange transfusion and up to five days for topping up. Some centres use plasma reduced CPD blood less than four hours old for exchange transfusion as this contains a full complement of coagulation factors, viable platelets and white cells. The use of fresh heparinized blood obtained by syringe from 'walking donors', usually hospital staff, is not recommended as the risk of transmitting hepatitis B and CMV transmission is greater, and variable amounts of anticoagulant used may increase any haemorrhagic tendency present.

Transfusion for anaemia

The haemoglobin in neonates varies with age (Table 10.1) and the degree of anaemia should be assessed in relation to this, but it should

Table 10.1   Haemoglobin levels in children

Age Cord blood gestation (weeks)	Hb (g/dl)
28	14
32	15.5
36	16
Term	16.5
Peripheral blood	
1–3 days	18.5
1 week	17.5
2 weeks	16.5
1 month	14
2–6 months	11.5
6 months – 2 years	12
2–6 years	12.5
6–12 years	13.5
then adult values	

not be allowed to fall below about 9 g/dl. Packed red cells are usually used for topping-up transfusions and as a rule of thumb 10 ml of packed cells will raise the haemoglobin of a normal, 3.5 kg, newborn by about 1 g/dl.

Haemolytic disease of the newborn

Haemolytic disease of the newborn (HDN) is caused by a blood group difference between the fetus and the mother. Most blood groups can be involved but the most common and severe cases are caused by differences in the rhesus blood group system, the mother being rhesus negative (dd) while the fetus is rhesus positive carrying the D-antigen (Dd or DD).

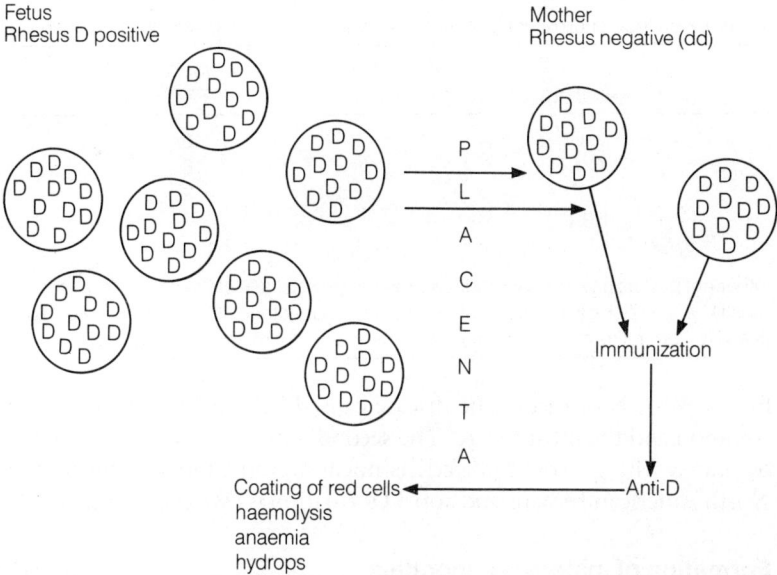

Fig. 10.1 In haemolytic disease of the newborn fetal cells pass across the placenta and immunize the mother. The anti-D produced passes back to the fetus lysing the fetal red cells and causing HDN.

The mechanism of the disease is outlined in Fig. 10.1. During delivery sufficient fetal red cells cross the placenta and enter the maternal circulation to immunize the mother producing antibodies to any blood group differences between the fetus and the mother. Any IgG antibodies produced will pass across the placenta in a subsequent pregnancy, coating the red cells of the fetus. Later such coated cells will be haemolysed in the fetus causing anaemia. After birth a positive direct antiglobulin test is found, an increase in unconjugated bilirubin occurs and this can give rise to kernicterus if it exceeds certain levels (page 162).

Treatment of HDN, when indicated, consists of replacing the fetal red cells by exchange transfusion with red cells which will not react with any antibody present and therefore will not be haemolysed. In practice the blood to be given is chosen so as not to carry any antigens to which the mother has made antibodies. In other respects the cells should match those of the fetus in the usual way.

The frequency of antibodies detected during pregnancy is given in Table 10.2. The rhesus antibodies are the most important and account

Table 10.2   Incidence of antibodies causing haemolytic disease of the newborn

Antibody	Incidence (%)
D	40
C + D	18
E	9
K(Kell)	6
c, Cw, D + E, c + E, e, Wr^a	2–5 each

Other antibodies have rarely produced haemolytic disease of the newborn; this is mostly very mild: Kpa, Fya, Fyb, M, S, Bga, Lua, Lub, other MNSs system antibodies, Jka, Jkb, as well as other extremely rare antibodies (for review see Beal, 1979).

for about 90% of cases. The disease caused by anti-D is still the most common and the most severe. The second most severe disease is caused by anti-c. The genotype cde/cde is not found in Chinese, Japanese or North American Indians and anti-D formation is extremely rare.

Formation of maternal antibodies

The formation of antibodies in the mother depends on the dose of the fetal cells. When large amounts of D-positive blood are given by transfusion to rhesus negative individuals up to 80% form antibodies; with smaller amounts only about 20% form antibodies. For these individuals only 0.5 ml are sufficient to cause antibody formation. During normal pregnancy it is difficult to detect fetal red cells in the maternal circulation and these are usually insufficient to cause antibody formation. During delivery and abortion large numbers of fetal cells cross the placenta; detectable numbers of cells also cross the placenta during obstetric manipulation of the fetus, in the presence of retroplacental bleeding and antepartum haemorrhage. In these situations antibody formation occurs in about 20% of cases and they should be monitored, prophylactic measures being taken when indicated (page 160). There is some variation in the antigenicity of D according to the genotype of the fetus and Du is a less potent antigen.

A significant factor which affects the number of fetuses sensitized is the ABO compatibility of the fetal blood *vis-à-vis* that of the mother. For example, if the mother has anti-A and the fetus is group A, then the chance of forming anti-D is much smaller. The reasons for this are not clear but it may be due to the more rapid destruction of the red cells in these individuals or because their destruction follows a different pathway (Fig. 10.2). On this basis it was postulated that the injection of anti-D would remove D-positive cells rapidly from the

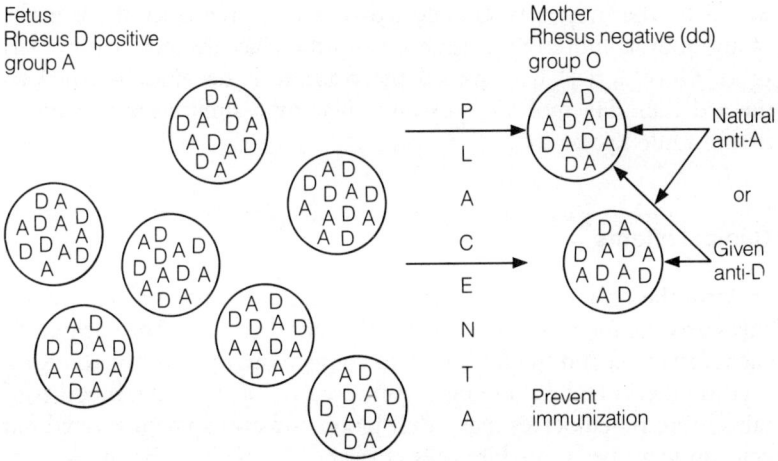

Fig. 10.2 If the mother has circulating antibodies to the fetal red cells, these will be destroyed and immunization will be prevented, thus preventing the occurrence of HDN.

circulation and prevent the formation of anti-D. This procedure forms the basis of the prevention of haemolytic disease of the newborn due to anti-D (page 160).

Previous exposure to D-positive cells

Previous exposure to D-positive cells by blood transfusion, certain blood products, or pregnancy including abortions will make the formation of clinically significant amounts of antibody more likely. Therefore in such cases about 20% of fetuses will have haemolytic disease of the newborn during the first pregnancy, while without previous sensitization this is extremely rare.

Transplacental passage of antibodies

Only IgG can cross the placenta, but this is quite slow taking several weeks to equilibrate. However, if the fetus is D-positive, the rate of transfer is more rapid as some of the antibody is removed from the fetal plasma by the fetal red cells. Anti-D can cross the placenta in the first trimester and even destroy red cells at this stage; such fetuses would be the most severely affected. Later in pregnancy the transfer of antibody is more rapid. IgG1 crosses the placenta more easily than IgG3. Once anti-D has crossed the placenta it becomes attached to the red cells. Haemolysis is extravascular by a similar mechanism to that in adults (page 124).

Clinical effects

In utero the only effect of antibody coating is haemolysis. The earlier this starts the more severely affected the fetus becomes. The haemolysis causes anaemia and the fetus tries to compensate for this by producing erythropoietin and expanding erythropoiesis. Normal fetal blood contains more reticulocytes than adult blood and also some nucleated red cell (up to 10 per 100 white cells at birth). As the fetus becomes more anaemic the number of nucleated red cells in the blood increases, hence the name erythroblastosis fetalis. When the degree of anaemia gets more severe the fetus suffers from cardiac failure and becomes oedematous with ascites, namely hydrops fetalis. It was thought that the liver in these cases was also affected and low plasma proteins contributed to the formation of the oedema. Because hydrops can be reversed by transfusion in utero it is probably mainly due to the anaemia. The most severely affected fetuses die *in utero*. Before birth the placenta clears any bilirubin from the fetal blood and jaundice at birth is usually only mild.

After birth the haemolysis of the baby's cells continues until any maternal antibody has been used up and the anaemia often becomes severe. More importantly the unconjugated bilirubin level can rise to levels that can cause kernicterus and this can be prevented by exchange transfusion (page 159).

Management of the sensitized pregnancy

With the wide availability of suitable panels of genotyped red cells all pregnant women are screened for the presence of antibodies and this would not only detect anti-D, but also any other atypical antibodies indicating the possibility of haemolytic disease of the newborn due to other antibodies. In very rare individuals in whom severe haemolytic disease of the new born is suspected because of the finding of fetal ascites by ultrasound, the disease may be due to a 'private antigen' carried by the father. In these the diagnosis can be made by reacting the father's red cells with the maternal serum (after absorption of any complicating naturally occurring maternal antibodies if indicated). Once an antibody has been discovered it must be identified (page 213). Antibodies in the mother should be tested for routinely as in Table 10.3.

Table 10.3   Antibody screening in pregnant rhesus-negative women

All mothers	test at 12 weeks
Negative antibody screen	first pregnancy retest at 28 and 34 weeks later pregnancies retest 8-weekly retest all at delivery
Positive antibody screen	retest at 16, 20, 24, 28 weeks, then 2-weekly

The genotype of the father is also important because if, for example, he is Dd then the fetus has a 50% chance of being rhesus negative (dd) and will be unaffected.

The severity of the disease in the fetus

Before birth the severity of the disease is assessed by the amount or titre of antibody in the maternal blood, the history of previous pregnancies, the bile pigment (bilirubin) level in the amniotic fluid, and findings on ultrasound examination.

ANTIBODY TITRE IN MATERNAL BLOOD

Rising levels of antibody indicate an affected fetus and amniocentesis would be indicated at levels above 4 µg/ml or a titre of 1:16 or above. This is of greatest value in the first pregnancy. If high levels are present early in pregnancy, ultrasound monitoring should be started at 16 weeks to detect the appearance of fetal ascites. The level of antibody found in the mother correlates badly with the severity of the disease in the fetus and a drop in maternal antibody levels from previously high levels is not a sign of a better outcome. Recent work suggests that measurement of opsonizing potential of the antibodies may be a better predictor of the severity of HDN than the titre of antibody.

HISTORY OF PREVIOUS PREGNANCIES

In first affected infants the disease tends to be mild and only 6% are stillborn if allowed to go to term. If severe disease is suspected on antibody levels then there is usually a history of previous sensitization. In second affected fetuses the disease is more severe and about 30% would be stillborn if allowed to go to term. In later pregnancies the severity of the disease often does not change but in some cases the fetus can be much more severely affected. Therefore a history of a previously affected infant is an indication for monitoring by ultrasound from 16 weeks onward at weekly intervals and by amniocentesis after 25 weeks gestation. Antibody titres are not reliable.

BILE PIGMENT LEVELS IN AMNIOTIC FLUID

Amniocentesis is carried out on the indications outlined above to measure the amniotic fluid bile pigments. The sample is sent to the laboratory in a brown bottle to prevent degradation of the pigments by light and the level measured spectrophotometrically at 450 μm. The usual biochemical methods are not used because several different pigments are present. The results can only be interpreted after the 25th week of pregnancy. As the optical density falls during pregnancy the gestational age has to be taken into account (Fig. 10.3). The area above the top line indicates a severely affected fetus with a high chance of intrauterine death. If the pregnancy is over 33 weeks, induction of labour is indicated with treatment after delivery. If less than 33 weeks, intrauterine transfusion is used to tide the infant over until delivery can be safely carried out. In the grey area repeat examinations are carried out at two-weekly intervals; a rising bilirubin indicates a severely affected infant requiring treatment. In the bottom area repeat examinations are carried out as in Table 10.3.

ULTRASOUND EXAMINATION

Ultrasound is used to detect ascites in the fetus after the 16th week of pregnancy and in patients with high antibody levels early in pregnancy,

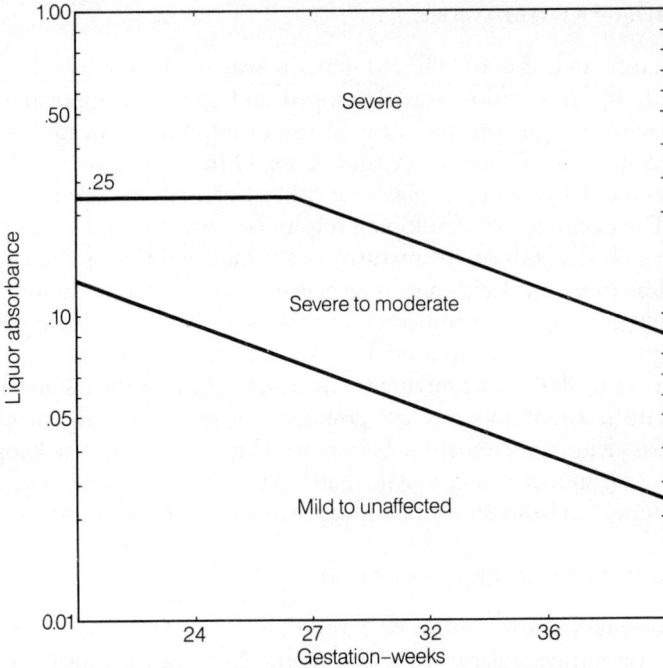

Fig. 10.3 Chart for the prediction of the severity of haemolytic disease of the newborn from amniotic fluid bilirubin; measurements expressed as absorbance at 450 nm.

or a history of a previously affected infant, it is made at weekly intervals until the 25th week when amniocentesis can be carried out. The finding of ascites indicates severe fetal anaemia indicating the need for intrauterine transfusion by fetoscopy.

Antenatal treatment of haemolytic disease of the newborn

Haemolytic disease of the newborn is not only treated after the baby is born, but successful therapy is available antenatally:

1 Early induction of labour.
2 Intrauterine transfusion.
3 Removal of antibodies from the maternal blood by plasmapheresis.

As each of these carries some risk for either the mother or the fetus it is important only to carry these out in sufficiently severely affected cases as outlined above.

PREMATURE DELIVERY

Premature delivery of affected fetuses was well established before intrauterine transfusion was developed and gave the opportunity of post-delivery treatment to fetuses at risk of intrauterine death between the 32nd week of pregnancy and term. Other less severely affected fetuses are delivered later when the risks of prematurity are very much less. The likelihood of developing respiratory distress syndrome (RDS) postnatally depends on the maturity of the lung and this can be assessed by measuring the lecithin/sphingomyelin ratio in the amniotic fluid. A value greater than 2 indicates a smaller chance of developing RDS. The presence of phosphotidyl-glycerol also indicates a sufficiently mature lung. These measurements are usually made at the last intrauterine transfusion at 29–30 weeks gestation, or just before the proposed time of delivery. Premature babies weighing more than a kilogram have, with modern care, a 95% chance of survival and the weight can be determined from ultrasound measurement of the abdominal girth.

INTRAUTERINE TRANSFUSION

Intrauterine transfusion can be carried by two techniques, intraperitoneally or intravascularly using fetoscopy. For both group O, rhesus negative (cde/cde) packed cells are used unless another blood group antibody is present in the mother. The donor cells should be cross-matched to the mother's serum. Intraperitoneal transfusion can only be used after the 24th week of pregnancy. The red cells rapidly enter the fetal circulation. The amount given is calculated by the formula (gestational age -20) $\times$ 10 ml packed cells. Unfortunately there is up to 40% fetal death with intraperitoneal transfusions. Intravascular transfusion can be carried out after the 18th week of pregnancy under direct vision by fetoscopy. The intrauterine haemoglobin can be measured before and after transfusion giving a reliable estimate of the severity of the disease. Repeat transfusions are given at two-weekly intervals. It is probable that intravascular transfusion has a lower fetal mortality compared to the intraperitoneal technique. Both these techniques require considerable obstetric skill and are only carried out in certain centres. The baby is delivered at about 32 to 34 weeks of pregnancy.

PLASMAPHERESIS

Plasmapheresis to remove maternal antibody is used for cases which have high antibody levels early in pregnancy, particularly in women with a previously severely affected infant. The efficacy of plasma exchange is doubtful and the fetus should in any case be carefully monitored by ultrasound and amniocentesis (see above). In order to be at all successful a 2 volume (*c*. 10 l) exchange should be carried out three times weekly starting at 10 or 12 weeks gestation. The plasma used should be from D-negative individuals because any D-positive red cell stroma stimulates further antibody formation.

Treatment of haemolytic disease of the newborn

In severely affected infants with gross anaemia or oedema (hydrops) immediate exchange transfusion is essential without waiting for laboratory results as suitable blood (group O compatible to the mother) can be ready before delivery.

Less severely affected neonates are investigated prior to treatment. In all cases the diagnosis is confirmed by a positive direct antiglobulin test. The best indicator of the severity of the disease is the haemoglobin level in the *cord* blood, the level of bilirubin and numbers of nucleated red cells being useful additional information. The normal cord blood haemoglobin is 14–20 g/dl at term, but is lower in premature infants (Table 10.1). Any haemoglobin value below 12.5 g/dl indicates an infant requiring exchange transfusion. A bilirubin above 60 μmol/l and a nucleated red cell count above 10 per 100 white cells would be further evidence of significant disease. The decision to exchange an infant with borderline disease depends on its clinical state. Prematurity, acidosis and a general poor condition are factors favouring exchange transfusion.

For exchange transfusion group O red cells not carrying any antigen to which the mother has made an antibody are used. This information should be available from the antenatal tests. Thus for most cases, i.e. anti-D, anti-D + C or anti-D + E, rhesus negative donor blood (cde/cde) is satisfactory, but, if anti-c or other antibody is present, the blood must be chosen accordingly. The donor cells must be cross-matched against the maternal and infant's sera. Fresh CPD blood is used (page 50). A 2 volume exchange (weight in kg × 90 × 2 ml) is used. Exchange transfusion not only corrects any anaemia present, but removes the infants antibody coated red cells which would eventually be destroyed and replaces these with red cells which will not be affected by the antibodies present. It also removes some unbound antibody and reduces the bilirubin level. It is easier to exchange at birth and prevent hyperbilirubinaemia than to treat it as it occurs. This is because bilirubin equilibrates between the extravascular space and plasma, and exchange transfusion is a relatively inefficient method of removal. Exchange transfusion, however, carries certain risks (Table 10.4) and should only be carried out for definitive indications.

Table 10.4   Risks of exchange transfusion

Cardiac arrhythmias or arrest
Circulatory overload or hypovolaemia
Necrotizing enterocolitis
Thrombosis, air emboli or perforation of vessels, excess anticoagulation,
    thrombocytopenia

After exchange transfusion the bilirubin in the plasma of the infant may still rise to unacceptable levels in which case further exchange transfusions may be indicated (see page 163). Finally, if the haemoglobin level drops below 9 g/dl, the infant may need a topping-up transfusion.

Prevention of haemolytic disease of the newborn

Rhesus negative, premenopausal females should not be given rhesus positive blood or blood products in all but exceptional circumstances.

The use of anti-D to prevent HDN

Shortly after the discovery that HDN was mainly due to anti-D it was noticed that the incidence of sensitization in mothers was reduced if they had had an ABO incompatible first pregnancy. This was thought to be due to the rapid removal of any fetal cells which had crossed the placenta. It was then postulated that, if fetal cells which had crossed the placenta could be destroyed rapidly, HDN would be prevented. As the largest number of fetal cells in the maternal circulation are found after delivery anti-D was given then to unsensitized mothers at risk. This prevented sensitization and greatly reduced the incidence of HDN in the next pregnancy. This method of preventing HDN is now more than 90% effective.

About 25 μg anti-D is needed to 'neutralize' a 1 ml transplacental haemorrhage (TPH), which is equivalent to fetal cell count in the mother of 1 per 2,400 maternal cells. The fetal cell count is made on the mother's blood using the 'Kleihauer test'. This depends on the finding that at acid pH Hb-A is eluted from the red cells while Hb-F is not, i.e.:

$$TPH = \frac{2,400 \times \text{number of fetal cells}}{\text{number of adult cells}} \, ml$$

After delivery of a rhesus positive child to a rhesus negative woman who has not been already sensitized, the mother is given 1 μg = 5 iu) anti-D IgG intravenously within 72 hours of delivery. In cases with large TPH the dose of anti-D is increased by 25 μg for every millilitre of TPH above one. This will prevent the occurrence of sensitization and subsequent HDN in most women at risk. However, some still become immunized and produce anti-D.

The reason for this is that there is some transplacental passage of fetal cells from the fetus to the maternal circulation at other times during pregnancy, mainly during threatened abortion, abortion, ectopic pregnancy, antepartum haemorrhage, concealed placental haemorrhage, obstetric manoeuvres such as amniocentesis, fetoscopy, version, etc. In such cases 50 μg of anti-D is given intravenously within 72 hours for events before the 20th week of pregnancy and 100 μg for events later. More is given if indicated by the fetal cell count. Even so some women still become immunized and this can probably be prevented by giving 100 μg anti-D i.m. at 28 and 34 weeks gestation. This dose of anti-D is harmless to the fetus as IgG only crosses the placenta slowly. Although great care is taken a few women still 'slip through the net' and are not treated with anti-D.

HDN not due to anti-D

The severity of disease caused by the non-D antibodies is generally milder than that caused by anti-D, but ranges from very mild to cases with hydrops (Table 14.2). The management of a pregnancy and infant with this form of HDN is the same as that described for anti-D. Antibody identification is performed on maternal serum and standard antibody screens carried out on the mother antenatally will have already identified most.

HDN due to ABO incompatibility

The 'natural' IgM ABO antibodies found in the serum do not pass across the placenta and do not cause HDN, only high titre IgG anti-A or anti-B causing the disease. It mostly occurs in group O mothers.

However, not all infants of mothers with such antibodies will be affected, as the ABO antigens, although present, are not fully developed in the fetus. ABO incompatibility is usually only suspected after other causes of HDN have been excluded and the ABO difference between the infant and the mother is detected. The direct antiglobulin test on the fetal red cells is often negative or very weak. This is probably due to the low number of ABO antigenic sites on fetal red cells. The diagnosis is made by eluting the antibody (page 220) from the infant's red cells and showing its specificity against adult A or B cells or finding the antibody in the baby's plasma. The antibody is always IgG and lytic with added complement. The titre of the eluted antibody correlates with the severity of the disease in the infant. The disease is usually mild, but occasional patients will need transfusion. This should be with group O blood; in A or B adult blood the antigens are fully developed and such blood is more rapidly lysed than the baby's own cells. Any blood given should be cross-matched against maternal and infant's sera. The reason why mainly group O women develop IgG antibodies is not clear, but may be due to the near identity of the A and B antigens making it impossible for individuals of groups A, A_2 or B to provide help during a response to T dependent non-self antigens by B2 lymphocytes. Thus people of these groups are less able to produce immune IgG anti-ABO antibodies.

Maternal autoimmune haemolytic anemia

Another cause of haemolytic disease of the newborn is maternal autoimmune haemolytic anaemia. The disease varies from very mild to severe requiring early delivery and exchange transfusion. Exchange transfusion is particularly indicated as it will remove coated red cells and free antibodies. In some cases it will have to be repeated. The diagnosis may already be known but, if suspected, may easily be confirmed by performing a direct antiglobulin test on the maternal red cells.

Neonatal hyperbilirubinaemia

At birth the bilirubin conjugating enzymes, the glucuronyl transferases in the liver are present only in low concentrations and do not develop fully until some days after birth. Therefore unconjugated bilirubin accumulates in the plasma. This is particularly so in premature infants. When the amount of unconjugated bilirubin in the plasma is greater than about 300 μmol/l, it exceeds the amount that albumin can carry.

Bilirubin can then penetrate the blood–brain barrier. Because unconjugated bilirubin is fat-soluble it can enter neural cells, in particular the basal ganglia, such as the hippocampal cortex, the subthalamic nuclei as well as the cerebellum and lower auditory centres and cause kernicterus. Clinically this causes irreversible brain damage with spasticity, mental retardation and deafness and in some cases death. It is therefore important to keep the bilirubin at a safe level. This can be achieved to some degree with phototherapy which promotes oxidation of bilirubin to harmless derivatives. The enzyme can also be induced by certain drugs, such as phenobarbitone, which may be given to the mother before delivery, but this is rarely done. Even so in some infants the

Table 10.5   Level of unconjugated bilirubin at which exchange transfusion is indicated after the first 24 hours after birth

| Gestational age | Unconjugated bilirubin level for transfusion after the first day (μmol/l) | |
| | Infants | |
	'well'	'sick'
Less than 29 weeks	200	180
29–31 weeks	240	200
31–34 weeks	290	240
34–37 weeks	350	270
37 weeks and over	350	300

At birth a level higher than 60 μmol/l may indicate the need for exchange; during the first 24 hours, the levels indicating exchange are obtained by interpolating this level to those given above.

bilirubin level rises to dangerous levels (Table 10.5) and has to be removed by exchange transfusion.

Neonatal coagulation defects

Coagulation defects in neonates are treated by exchange transfusion using CPD blood less than four hours old, or with FFP. If FFP is used, the dose is 10 ml/kg, but care is necessary to avoid overloading the circulation. The indications for such replacement are different from those in adults and are beyond the scope of this book. In diagnosed haemophiliacs factor VIII concentrate can be used; cryoprecipitate is not used because of the volumes involved. Factor IX concentrate (PCC, page 107) has caused thrombosis and is not used.

Neonatal purpura

Platelet counts in the normal and premature neonate are similar to those in adults. The causes of neonatal thrombocytopenic purpura are given in Table 10.6. In general the indications for platelet replacement

Table 10.6   Causes of neonatal thrombocytopenia

Exchange transfusions
Maternal alloimmunization
Maternal autoimmunization (ITP)
Congenital infections
rubella
cytomegalovirus
toxoplasmosis
syphilis
bacterial
Giant hemangiomata
Absent radii

are the same as in adults (page 84) but a minimum level of $30 \times 10^9/l$ is taken. In calculating the dose care has to be taken not to use too big a volume and overload the circulation. The platelets may be gently spun down and excess plasma removed just before giving. Neonatal purpura due to maternal antibody is discussed on page 31.

Graft versus host disease

This occurs rarely in immune-compromised infants, particularly after granulocyte transfusion, and can be prevented by irradiating any blood prior to transfusion.

Further reading

Walker, W (1971) Haemolytic disease of the newborn. In: *Recent Advances in Paediatrics 4th Ed.*, p 119 Eds. Gairdner, D, Hull, D. J A Churchill, London.

Stockman, J. A (1983) The anaemia of prematurity and the decision when to transfuse. *Advances in Paediatrics*, 30, 191.

Beal, R. W (1979) Non-rhesus (D) blood group iso-immunisation in obstetrics. *Clinics in Obstetrics and Gynecology*, 6, 493.

Davey, M. (1979) The prevention of rhesus-isoimmunisation. *Clinics in Obstetrics and Gynecology*, **6**, 509.

Kay, L A (1984) Cellular basis of immune response to antigen of the ABO blood-group system. *Lancet*, **ii**, 1369.

11 Bone marrow transplantation

When a vital organ becomes so diseased that life is endangered, transplantation of a healthy organ from another individual may be considered if a suitable donor can be found.

The transplantation of solid organs is limited by the supply of suitable organs since in most cases it must be obtained in a suitable condition from a cadaver. Prevention of degenerative diseases and the development of artificial organs will in the long term become the most practical means of reducing the demand for solid organs for transplantation.

Fortunately marrow is a self-regenerative tissue and, apart from the need for a general anaesthetic, its donation does not compromise the health of the donor. Bone marrow transplantation (BMT) is being used in an increasing number of disorders as the problems associated with its use are overcome.

The principles of transplantation immunology

Rejection of the transplant

Only tissue from syngeneic individuals (monozygotic twins) will fail to evoke an immune response on transplantation. All nucleated cells bear HLA ABC determined class I molecules. These make them the target of host cytotoxic T cell responses, when transplanted into an allogeneic individual (Chapter 4). This may occur even between HLA ABC and D identical MLC negative siblings so that as yet undefined antigenic differences must also influence graft survival. For this reason all transplant recipients, except identical twins, receive immunosuppressive treatment to prevent graft rejection.

Graft versus host disease

Bone marrow itself contains immunocompetent cells and their precursors. T helper lymphocytes of the donor are activated by HLA class II molecules on the recipient cells, while alloreactive cytotoxic T lymphocytes are primarily directed against class I molecules. These interactions result in graft versus host disease (GVHD) in the immunocompromised recipient. GVHD is a greater problem than rejection in bone marrow transplantation. This is because the conditioning regimens not only ablate the myeloid/erythroid elements of the bone marrow but also provide powerful immune suppression in the host, making graft rejection unlikely. A degree of graft versus host disease has some benefits. It increases immune suppression of the host, improves marrow engraftment and may also have a graft versus leukaemia effect.

The effects of transfusion on the immunological response to the allograft

Prior transfusions may affect the likelihood of rejection by exposing the individual to HLA antigens on contaminating leucocytes. Depending on the volume and timing of blood transfusion and on the immunocompetence of the recipient, the effect may be beneficial or detrimental. In general:

1 Blood and blood products from potential donors should not be used.
2 Patients with leukaemia are grossly immunocompromised and unlikely to be sensitized by transfusion.
3 Patients with chronic renal failure are moderately immunocompromised but may be sensitized if large volumes (over 10 units) of blood are given making renal graft rejection more likely. However, the transfusion of smaller volumes of blood from unrelated donors in the six months before transplantation reduces graft rejection as explained in Chapter 4.

Bone marrow transplantation

The principles of the transplantation procedure are outlined in Fig. 11.1. Bone marrow transplantation is carried out for the treatment of leukaemia, lymphomas and other drug sensitive tumours to allow the use of tumour ablative doses of x-rays or cytotoxic drugs, for the replacement of marrow in severe aplastic anaemia and for the replacement of marrow in thalassaemia major and some inherited enzyme

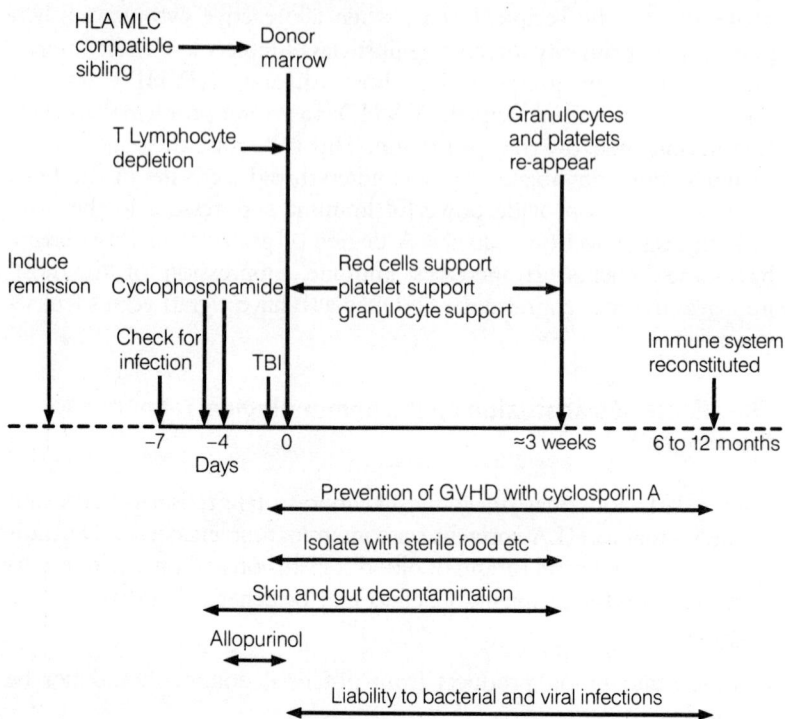

Fig. 11.1   Outline of bone marrow transplantation in acute leukaemia.

deficiencies. The results of transplantation above the age of 30–40 years have not been good because the severity of GVHD increases with age and in general bone marrow transplantation is limited to individuals below the age of 35 years.

Indications for bone marrow transplantation

Acute myeloid leukaemia

Despite advances in chemotherapy which have increased the remission rate to around 80%, the median duration of first remission is still only about 12 months, and response to further chemotherapy is very disappointing. If a suitable donor is available and transplantation is carried out early in first remission, a five-year survival with probable cure can be expected in up to 50% of individuals. The relapse rate in first remission transplants is about 20% occurring mostly in the first 12 months.

The maintenance of remission is also helped by a graft versus leukaemia effect. Transplantation in relapse fails in over 95% of patients and transplantation in second remission only gives a plateau of long-term survivors of 20–30%. These low success rates are due to relapse of the original disease.

Acute lymphoblastic leukaemia

Childhood acute lymphoblastic leukaemia in the good prognosis groups responds very well to conventional chemotherapy with a 70–80% chance of long-term survival. Transplantation in these is only indicated in relapsed cases during second (or subsequent) remission. Children in poor prognosis groups (with an initial blast cell count above 25×10^9 or T or B cell types) and adults in first remission also benefit from bone marrow transplantation.

Chronic myeloid leukaemia

In chronic granulocytic leukaemia transplantation in the chronic phase gives prolonged disease-free survival in about 75% of patients. In the accelerated phase results are not as good as in the chronic phase of the disease but are still useful. In blast crisis or in remission following blast crisis BMT is followed by early relapse in the majority of cases. Because of this it is important to arrange transplantation quickly so that patients do not go into blast crisis while on the waiting list.

Other malignancies

Marrow transplantation may allow sufficiently intense chemotherapy to eradicate myeloma or lymphoma failing to respond to conventional treatment, but experience is limited as most patients with these diseases are too old for the procedure.

Aplastic anaemia

Severe aplastic anaemias with platelets less than 10×10^9/l, granulocytes less than 0.5×10^9/l and severe anaemia, have a greater than 70% mortallity at five years with conventional treatment and a considerably better survival is achieved with bone marrow transplantation. Patients who have had prior blood transfusion are more likely to reject their transplants than those who have not been transfused, and early transplantation is recommended. If patients need transfusions or platelet support, they should be given washed, filtered red cells (page 56) and platelets with low granulocyte contamination (page 181). There appears to be some improvement in graft take if marrow donor buffy coat cells are given at the time of grafting to multiply transfused patients. Cyclosporin given for GVHD prophylaxis also decreases the proportion of grafts rejected, when compared with methotrexate. Other studies indicate that more intensive conditioning regimens than cyclophosphamide alone including total body irradiation reduce graft rejection, but have an increased mortality from complications.

Recently some good results in the treatment of severe aplastic anaemia have been obtained using anti-lymphocyte serum (ALG) and a prospective trial comparing this form of treatment with bone marrow transplantation is being carried out. However, blood product support is still required by over 30% of the survivors after one year of this treatment.

Congenital defects

Certain congenital enzyme deficiencies (Table 11.1), severe combined immunodeficiency and osteopetrosis may be corrected by marrow transplantion. This is done as early as possible before the complications of the disease become irreversible.

Table 11.1   Inherited conditions for which bone marrow transplantation has been used with some success

Severe combined immune deficiency syndrome (SCID)
β-thalassaemia major
Osteopetrosis
Wiskott-Aldrich syndrome
Various granulocyte disorders
Diamond-Blackfan syndrome
Fanconi's anaemia
Various mucopolysaccharidoses
Lipidosis
Gaucher's disease

In β-thalassaemia major bone marrow transplantation in patients under the age of about five years can cure the disease. However, as other treatment is available the 30% procedure related mortality has to be justified. In older patients with significant iron overload the procedure related mortality is even higher.

Bone marrow processing

Bone marrow processing is necessary for the following reasons:

1 To remove red cells in ABO incompatible transplantation.
2 To remove T lymphocytes to prevent graft versus host disease.
3 In autologous bone marrow transplantation it is used for volume reduction prior to freezing and also for purging of malignant cells if such techniques are available.

All marrow processing is, as far as possible, carried out in closed systems or in a laminar air flow cabinet to minimize the risk of introducing infection. The necessary procedures are outlined in Fig. 11.2.

Principles of the transplantation procedure

Selection of bone marrow donor

Histocompatibility is of great importance in preventing GVHD in bone marrow transplantation. In transplantation between identical twins (syngeneic) there is complete identity and GVHD is not a problem. Although the relapse rate in leukaemia is higher in syngeneic transplants, the procedure related mortality is lower and these donors are still the first choice. Otherwise HLA (A, B, D) identical, MLC negative donors are used if available. Sibling donors with one haplotype match and differing only at either the A or B locus with a negative MLC have also given good results. Transplantation with a greater degree of mismatch has so far not given satisfactory results because of the occurrence of severe GVHD (page 174). If a sibling or other relative with the required match is not available, then a suitable match may be searched for using a panel of volunteer donors. However, it is too early to know whether unrelated, HLA AB D matched MLC negative donors give the same results as related donors.

The donor is given a full clinical examination and a unit of blood is taken to replace the blood loss (1 l) during the harvest procedure.

ABO incompatibility

ABO incompatibility does not affect the outcome of bone marrow transplantation. The bone marrow donation is depleted of the incompatible

Infuse into recipient ◄——— HARVEST IL BONE MARROW
after filtering

◄—— Volume reduction on haemonetics cell
separator removing excess plasma
and 75% of red cells

240 ml

Storage in liquid nitrogen; for
autologous BMT the marrow is frozen
in a programmed freezer after the
addition of DMSO (marrow: DMSO 3:1)

Red cell removal by sedimentation after
◄—— the addition of hydroxy-ethyl starch
(marrow: HES 5:1); wash ×2 with RPMI

Thaw at 37°C and return to patient   Red cell poor marrow

Removal of T-lymphocytes or other   ABO incompatible BMT
unwanted cells with either
(i) specific antibody/complement lysis
(ii) specific antibody directed toxin
(ricin A-chain) or
(iii) specific antibody using a second
layer on a solid matrix (magnetic
beads) to physically remove cells

Wash ×2 with RPMI

Infuse to recipient

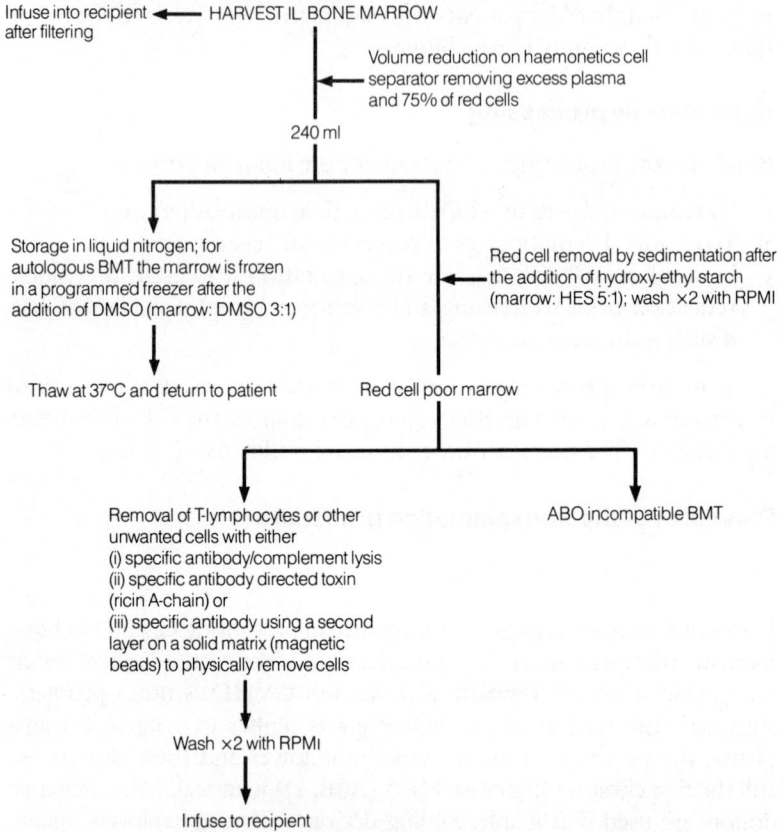

Fig. 11.2   Outline of bone marrow processing.

red cells, and the recipient may also be plasma-exchanged to reduce
high titre ABO antibodies in his blood.

Marrow harvest

The marrow is obtained under general anaesthesia by multiple aspira-
tion from the iliac crests and sternum. A minimum of 2×10^8 cells
per kg recipient weight will be needed to reconstitute marrow function
and for adults about 1 litre has to be taken. The marrow is collected

into ACD or preservative free heparin anticoagulant and is given via a standard blood filter (170 μm) to remove clumps of cells.

The conditioning regimen

Before the donor marrow can be given to the patient he is prepared by a conditioning regimen designed to treat any residual malignant disease, ablate the bone marrow and 'create space' and destroy the immune system so that the foreign marrow can take.

In acute myeloid leukaemia high dose cyclophosphamide (60 mg/kg/day) is given on days −5 and −4 followed by total body irradiation (TBI) (10 Gy on day −1). The actual dose, rate and number of fractions given varies between centres. In the treatment of CGL and ALL slight variations of the above scheme are recommended by different centres and special regimens have been devised for other malignancies.

In severe aplastic anaemia high dose cyclophosphamide, 50 mg/kg/day on four successive days, are given to achieve graft take, but this is not always successful. Some centres add procarbazine and anti-lymphocyte globulin or sublethal doses of TBI or total lymphoid irradiation to increase the chance of marrow take. Giving buffy coat prepared from the marrow donor for the five days after the transplant decreases the rejection rate and increases the survival of patients in aplastic anaemia.

In the inherited diseases TBI is not used. The aim is to use the minimum amounts of cytotoxic drugs to allow graft take. The most successful scheme is to give busulphan, 20 mg/kg, followed by cyclophosphamide, 50 mg/kg/day, on four successive days. Lower doses have been followed by regrowth of recipient marrow.

Engraftment

The donor marrow is infused into a peripheral vein, stem cells develop in the marrow 'microenvironment' to reconstitute haematopoeisis including the production of T and B lymphocytes. Granulocytes and platelets reappear in the blood after two to three weeks or even longer, the platelets appearing later. Immunological responsiveness is reconstituted more slowly over 12 months. T helper cells appear later than other cells and there is a prolonged defect in humoral immunity. This and the defect in cellular immunity is more marked in patients with GVHD.

Problems: prevention and management

Radiation and drug toxicity

Radiotherapy results in oropharyngeal mucositis, may also affect other organs and predisposes to pneumonitis. Fractionation of the dose may reduce toxicity. Cyclophosphamide causes haemorrhagic cystitis which is prevented by adequate hydration and treatment with mesna which prevents appearance of a toxic metabolite in the urine. The major effect of the regime is immunosuppression.

Graft versus host disease (GVHD)

Graft versus host disease is caused by donor T lymphocytes reacting against antigens of the host tissues. It is classified into acute GVHD and chronic GVHD. These can occur independently or merge into each other. They tend to be more severe in older patients.

Acute GVHD occurs during the first 100 days after transplantation in 70% of matched recipients with a mortality of 20%. It starts with a maculopapular skin rash, which is often seen on the palms of the hands, and this may progress to a bullous eruption. There may be abdominal cramps and severe watery diarrhoea. Hepatic cellular necrosis and bile duct damage occur. It is classified into four grades of severity. Prevention of acute GVHD is by immune suppression with methotrexate or cyclosporin A. Both reduce the incidence and severity of the disease, but with cyclosporin, the disease is generally milder, and its use may allow quicker engraftment, but it has considerable renal toxicity. Another factor affecting the severity of acute GVHD is the occurrence of bacterial or viral infections.

More recently GVHD has been prevented by the removal of T lymphocytes from the marrow using mouse monoclonal antibodies before grafting, but in some individuals this has caused graft failure. However, as these techniques improve it may be possible to graft in the presence of an HLA mismatch, or using matched unrelated donors, making allogeneic bone marrow grafting available to many more individuals.

Treatment of established acute GVHD is with high dose methyl prednisolone, anti-lymphocyte globulin and increased doses of cyclosporin. Response is generally poor in severe cases.

Chronic graft versus host disease occurs 3–18 months after transplantation and affects up to 40% of patients. This may be related to minor (non-HLA) compatibility antigen mismatch. The condition ranges from a mild localized rash to a multisystem disease resembling various autoimmune diseases affecting the liver, lungs, skin, etc. There is also profound immune paresis. Treatment is by immune suppression with prednisone, cyclophosphamide, procarbazine or azathioprine over a period of time.A serious complication is pneumococcal septicaemia.

Infection

Early in the post-transplant period before engraftment, bacterial infections are the major problem. As in all immune-suppressed patients organisms such as *Pseudomonas*, other Gram-negative bacteria, anaerobes and staphylococci are encountered, often derived from the patient rather than the environment.

To prevent such infections arising the patient receives skin and gut decontamination, and possible sites for infection are bacteriologically monitored. Nursing in laminar air flow rooms and sterile food prevent environmentally derived infection. Wide spectrum, high dose bactericidal antibiotics are given as soon as sustained fever develops.

Immunity to viral, fungal and other organisms is also compromised. Because of late recovery of T cell function, viral infection is a danger for several years post transplantation. CMV infection is particularly important and CMV antiglobulin is used prophylactically. Herpes zoster can be prevented by zoster immunoglobulin (page 117). Established herpes zoster and simplex infections respond to acyclovir and this is used prophylactically in some centres. Vaccination with live attenuated viruses is contraindicated.

A major problem occurring during the first three to nine months after bone marrow transplantation is interstitial pneumonitis. The pathogenesis of this condition is not entirely clear. It appears to be related to chronic GVHD, but TBI and CMV or other viral infections also play a part in its aetiology. Treatment is with steroids, but it is often fatal. Septrin prophylaxis prevents pneumocystis carinii pneumonitis.

Anaemia, granulocytopenia, thrombocytopenia

These occur in the weeks before engraftment is complete and are treated by replacement therapy in the usual way (Chapters 5, 6, 7). CMV negative donors are used for a CMV negative patient with a CMV negative graft if possible. All blood products are irradiated to 15Gy before use.

Recurrence of the original disease

Aplastic anaemia may not be corrected by marrow transplantation, and it is speculated that the defect in marrow 'microenvironment' causing the original disease may prevent engraftment.

Leukaemia relapse is more likely to occur after syngeneic transplantation than after allogeneic transplantation. Recurrence of leukaemia in the donor type cells has also been reported and occurs in about 7% of relapses.

Autologous bone marrow transplantation

Autologous bone marrow transplantation (ABMT) is used to enable the administration of supralethal chemotherapy or radiotherapy in an attempt to eradicate certain malignant diseases. However, it has to be remembered that ABMT only combats the marrow toxicity of drugs and doses are still limited by effects on other tissues. The conditions treated have been leukaemias, lymphomas and certain other solid tumours.

Acute leukaemia

In acute leukaemia the marrow used for autologous bone marrow transplantation is harvested during (first) remission. Formerly the harvested marrow was stored, and ablative chemotherapy or TBI with ABMT was given on relapse. Although most patients had a further remission only very few survived over two years. Similarly poor survival resulted if the procedure was used in second remission even if first remission stored marrow was used. Analysis of these results and comparison with syngeneic bone marrow transplantation indicated that relapse was largely due to failure to eradicate the disease in the patient at these stages of the disease rather than the infusion of leukaemic cells with the autologous marrow.

In order to increase the chance of eradicating residual leukaemic cells the procedure is now carried out in first remission. The patient is induced by standard chemotherapy and is then given consolidation chemotherapy. If the patient is eligible for allogeneic transplantation and has a donor, this would be the treatment of choice. For ABMT the same criteria as for allotransplantation are followed but, because the procedure is less traumatic and GVHD is not a problem, individuals up to 55–60 years old are eligible. The patient is prepared as for allografting, the marrow is harvested and stored in liquid nitrogen. The patient is then treated (conditioned) either with ablative chemotherapy or with cyclophosphamide and TBI. The stored marrow is then returned to the patient. During the aplastic phase which lasts about three weeks the patient is reverse barrier nursed.

In AML the results have been promising and up to 50% of patients have achieved long-term remissions. Because the numbers in each series with adequate follow up is still small no firm conclusions can be drawn. In ALL there are few results for ABMT in first remission but the technique does not look as promising as in AML, but purging with antibodies may be possible.

Bone marrow purging

Even in first remission the bone marrow probably contains some leukaemic cells and ABMT can only be curative if the bone marrow is treated to remove these before reinfusion. This can be done either with drugs that will kill leukaemic cells at lower concentrations than normal stem cells or by attacking the leukaemic cells with specific antibodies and lysing or removing them.

In AML no specific antibodies are available and several investigators have tried various drugs for *in-vitro* purging. There is no difference in *in-vitro* drug sensitivity between leukaemic and normal stem cells in culture and clinical results do not differ from those obtained with unpurged marrow.

In ALL suitable monoclonal antibodies are available for purging. One approach has been similar to the removal of T cells from marrow. The marrow is incubated with antibodies which are known to react with the malignant cells and is then treated with complement. Other investigators have conjugated the A-chain of ricin, a lethal toxin from plants, to a suitable monoclonal antibody. Another approach is to combine the antibody to magnetic beads and then use these to remove cells from the marrow. Considerable amount of work using this system has been done in neuroblastoma and in Burkitt's lymphoma with some promising results.

Another approach which is applicable to both AML and ALL in first remission is to use '*in-vivo* purging', which is achieved by a double autologous transplant. The ABMT procedure is repeated as soon as marrow regeneration has occurred after the first ABMT. It is believed that the normal cells will grow more rapidly than the leukaemic cells and that the number of leukaemic cells reinfused with the second marrow is extremely small.

Lymphoma

Patients with high grade non-Hodgkin's lymphoma without marrow involvement have been treated with high dose chemotherapy followed by autologous bone marrow transplantation with promising results. Prolonged remissions in patients with extensive poor prognosis disease have been produced with possible cure in some. As patients with these conditions respond well to conventional chemotherapy selection for ABMT is crucial, and for consideration patients should have failed to achieve complete remission after initial therapy. Some groups, for example, the British National Lymphoma Investigation, now consider that patients who fail to enter complete remission after three courses of intensive chemotherapy (CHOP) are eligible for ABMT, as well as those who relapse later.

In Hodgkin's disease there are even less data, but patients who fail to respond to second line therapy should be considered for ABMT as preliminary results look promising.

Other solid tumours

Neuroblastoma

Some long-term responses have been achieved in stage III and IV neuroblastoma. Contamination of the bone marrow by malignant cells is an important problem and purging using antibody directed magnetic beads is under investigation.

Small cell carcinoma of the lung

ABMT has only been applied to limited disease without marrow involvement. Although little prolongation of life has been achieved so far the morbidity of ABMT is considerably less than that of repeated courses of conventional chemotherapy and patients find it more tolerable. ABMT at present has only a limited role in this condition.

Other tumours which have been treated with high dose chemotherapy and ABMT with promising preliminary results are glioblastoma, testicular carcinoma and melanoma. ABMT may also be useful in ovarian cancer and Ewing's sarcoma; it does not appear to be helpful in carcinoma of the breast, where widespread metastasis of dormant cells occurs.

Further reading

Seminars in Haematology (1984) **24**, nos. 1, 2 and 3.

Nathan, D G (Ed.) (1984) Bone marrow transplantation. *Clinics in Haematology*, **12**, no. 3.

Goldstone, A H, Linch, D C (1985) Autologous bone marrow transplantation. *Clinics in Haematology*, **14**, no. 2.

12 Cell separation and plasma exchange

Cell separators are used in two main areas of medicine. The first is for the production of platelets, granulocytes and plasma by the blood transfusion service and this use of cell separators has already been described (Chapters 6, 7, 8). The second use is directly in the treatment of patients to remove unwanted, excess cells or replace plasma containing harmful constituents. All cell separators depend on centrifugation, which separates cellular components and plasma according to their relative densities. The addition of red cell sedimenting agents, such as hydroxyethyl starch (HES), which act by causing rouleaux formation, is necessary for the separation of granulocytes from red cells. Thus red cells are 'spun down' most rapidly followed closely by granulocytes and then lymphocytes. Platelets are slightly denser than plasma and come next, while plasma appears at the centre of the centrifuge bowl. Two types of cell separators have been developed. In one the centrifuge bowl is filled intermittently and the blood is processed batchwise, while in the other continuous flow processing is used. Plasma can also be separated from the cellular elements of the blood by filtration.

Intermittent flow cell separators

The intermittent cell separator system has mainly been developed by Haemonetics. In this system (Fig. 12.1) the blood is continuously anticoagulated as it is pumped into a spinning centrifuge bowl. The anticoagulant used is usually citrate based, but for some purposes preservative free heparin is used. As the blood enters the bowl the centrifugal force separates the various components and these can be drawn off sequentially into separate collecting bags. Finally the red cells from the bowl can be returned to the patient. In plasma exchange the removed plasma is replaced by the infusion of PPF, FFP or other replacement fluid (page 196). The whole system including the centrifuge bowl in contact with the blood is made from disposable plastics in various designs optimized for each specific purpose. These intermittent machines are easy to use and reliable. Recent specialized developments

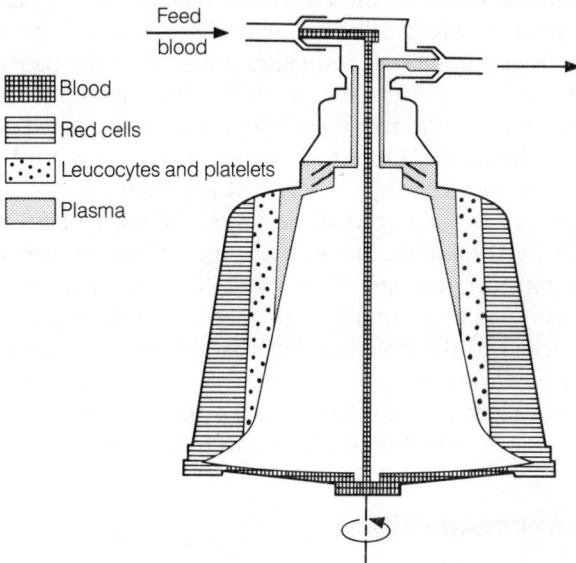

Fig. 12.1 The Haemonetics intermittent flow cell separator. Anticoagulated blood is pumped into the rotating bowl of the machine and plasma and cell separation begins as the bowl fills, the plasma being nearest the centre of the bowl, then the platelet layer, followed by the white cells and furthest out the red cells. When the bowl is full, as further blood is pumped in, the plasma is expelled followed by the platelets and white cells. These are collected as required. When the bowl is full of red cells, the centrifuge is stopped and uncollected elements are pumped to a bag for gravity reinfusion into the donor. The procedure is then repeated until enough 'components' have been collected. These machines are simple to operate and are used for platelet, granulocyte and plasma collection. (From Mollison, P L, 1983)

allow the harvesting of 2 units of plasma and 2–2.5×10^{11} platelets with minimal red and white cell contamination in a closed system. This is useful for the large scale harvesting of plasma by the blood transfusion service and the simultaneous production of single donor platelet packs.

Continuous flow cell separators

Continuous flow cell separators have been developed by several manu-facturers (IBM, Aminco, Travenol). The principle of these is that the blood is pumped continuously into the bottom of the centrifuge bowl and as the blood rises in the centrifuge chamber it is separated into layers of plasma, white cells and red cells. These can be separately and continuously drawn off and either returned to the patient or col-lected. Thus, if one is harvesting granulocytes, then only the fraction containing these is collected, the remaining plasma and red cells being returned to the donor. Once the machine is set up it can be run for as long as two or even three hours and large numbers of white cells or platelets can be harvested. Care has to be taken that the patient is not made hypovolaemic. Plasma exchange can be done very efficiently with this type of machine. The latest Travenol machine (Fenwal CS3000) (Fig. 12.2) is arranged so that a complete plastic harness can be attached to the machine. Two bags from this are put into the centrifuge bowl, one to separate the various blood components and the other to collect the required cells and concentrate them. This dimin-ishes the risks of hypovolaemia as the machine is running.

Plasma exchange filters

Plasma can be separated from the cellular elements of the blood by passing it over a filter with a pore size of approximately 0.2 μm. In such a system (Fig. 12.3) a considerable filter area must be available for the separation to be fast enough for clinical use. This has been achieved by the use of hollow fibre filters. The pressure gradient between the inside of the hollow filter must be just right for filtration of about 80% of the plasma to take place. The filter capsule and lines to the patient are all in one sterile unit. This is put into the purpose-designed pumping system, which automatically pumps the filtered plasma into a collecting bag and returns the cellular elements to the patient together with the desired amount of replacement fluid. The system has a low extracorporeal volume and hypovolaemia is generally not a problem.

Dangers associated with the use of cell separators

The use of cell separators to exchange or remove various blood compo-nents carries with it the dangers of both hypo- and hypervolaemia.

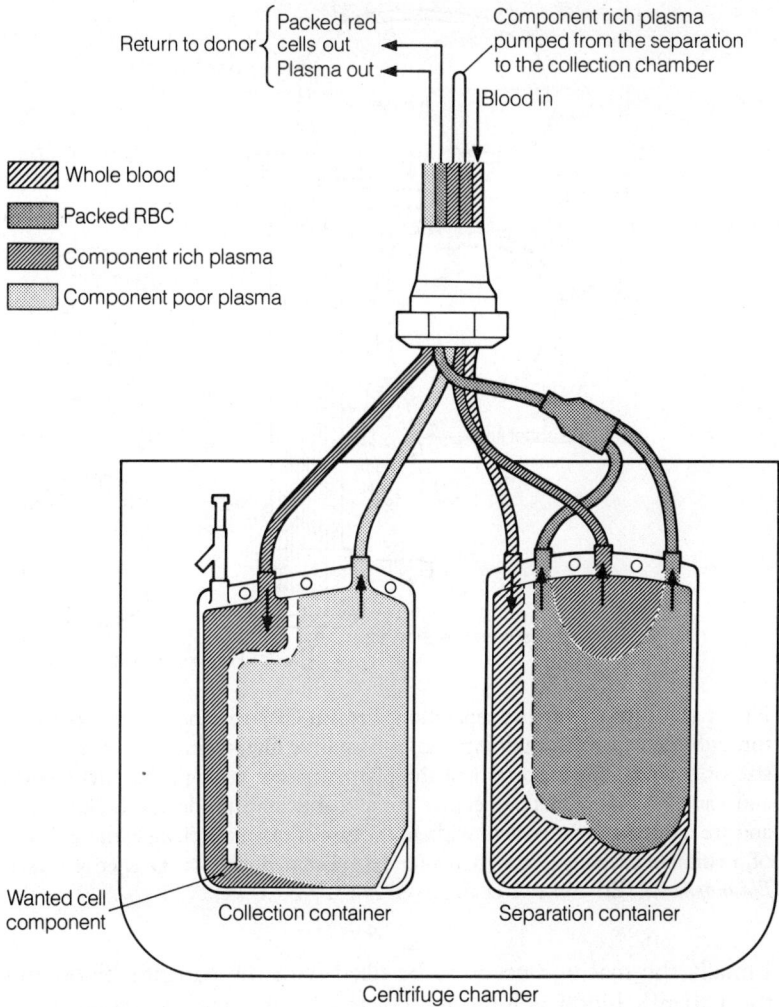

Fig. 12.2 The Fenwal CS-3000 continuous flow blood cell separator. The blood is pumped into the separation bag. This plastic bag is shaped by a former in the centrifuge head so that the middle outlet tube is nearest the centre of the centrifuge. The component-rich plasma passes out through this and is pumped into the collection bag. In this the desired cell component, platelets or white cells, are concentrated and collected. The plasma and the packed red cells are then returned to the patient.

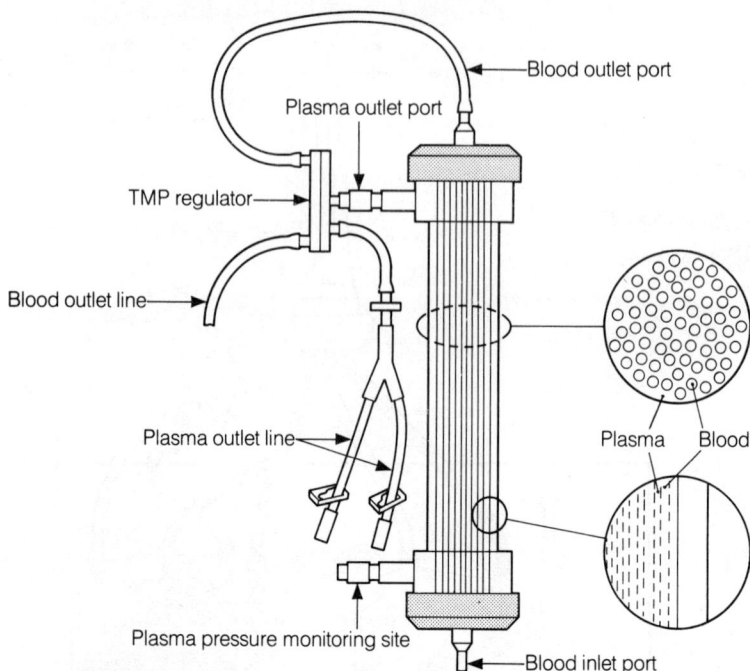

Fig. 12.3 Capillary plasma separation, Fenwal CPS-10. The blood is pumped through the capsule containing 800 hollow fibre filters with a maximum pore size of 0.55 μm. A proportion of the plasma passes through the filter's pores and can be collected. The cellular components stay inside the hollow filter and are returned to the patient with, in the case of plasma exchange, the addition of a suitable exchange fluid (Chapter 13). (From Buchholz, D L et al (1983), *Plasmapheresis*. Ed. Nose, Y et al. Raven Press, New York)

Initially the machine needs to be filled with the patient's blood and the patient's blood volume is depleted by the amount required for this. It is therefore important to use the correct size centrifugation chamber for the size of patient. It is also very important that exact records of the volumes removed and put back are kept as recommended by the manufacturer.

Other potential hazards are citrate toxicity, haemolysis and cardiac arrhythmias. The rapid infusion of cold fluid into the veins is a potential cause of the latter. Further hazards are those due to the venous access. It has to be remembered that the blood and fluid are pumped by the machine and great care has to be taken to avoid air embolism and the machines include 'bubble sensors' which, when activated, turn the machine off. Also the same infectious hazards exist in plasma exchange as with any other transfusions. A special hazard associated with plasma exchange, particularly if plasma substitutes are used, is the reduction of coagulation factors and immunoglobulins leading to bleeding and infection respectively. In plasma, granulocyte and platelet donors reduction of lymphocytes is a potential hazard and leads to lower but not abnormal immunoglobulin levels. The addition of sedimenting agents is also a potential hazard. HES is safe but causes prolonged itching in a few donors.

Red cell exchange

Red cell exchange is carried out in haemolytic disease of the newborn (Chapter 9) and sickle cell disease (page 68) and is best done manually.

In polycythaemia reduction of the haematocrit is important to decrease the blood viscosity. In primary polycythaemia and secondary polycythaemia due to abnormal erythropoietin production or high affinity haemoglobins (only indicated if the haematocrit is very high) simple, repeated venesection is sufficient. In patients with secondary polycythaemia due to cardiac and pulmonary disease, reducing the blood viscosity by venesection and increasing blood flow often makes the patient feel considerably better, although the oxygen delivery capacity by each millilitre of blood is reduced. In these patients great care has to be taken because even small reductions in blood volume may cause a reduction in cardiac output with fatal consequences and the blood volume is maintained by replacing any red cells removed with plasma or a plasma substitute. Again it is simpler to do this manually. Iron is given to these patients to prevent iron deficiency.

Iron overload not due to transfusion is also treated by manual venesection.

In very severe autoimmune haemolytic anaemia it may be useful to do an exchange transfusion. Plasma exchange would remove any antibodies present in the plasma, but as most antibodies are absorbed on the red cells a better result may be obtained if they are also removed. This form of treatment would only apply to the most severe cases not responding to other forms of therapy.

Platelet reduction

This is occasionally indicated in individuals with platelet counts over

1,000 × 10⁹/l due to a myeloproliferative disorder who have symptoms of thrombosis or bleeding. Platelet reduction has to be carried out daily for a few days until treatment of the underlying condition takes effect.

White cell reduction

Leukapheresis is used in *chronic granulocytic leukaemia* as initial treatment to reduce very high white counts before chemotherapy has had time to be effective. White cell aggregates tend to form when the WBC exceeds 150 × 10⁹/l and vascular occlusion in the microcirculation produces altered consciousness and other neurological abnormalities, pulmonary dysfunction, thrombosis, priapism and papilloedema. Leukapheresis rapidly reduces the white cell count and prevents and relieves these complications making the patient feel better. Initially the leukapheresis is carried out daily, but later every second or third day is enough to keep the total WBC below 50 × 10⁹/l. Long-term therapy by leukapheresis does not affect the course of the disease and should not replace conventional treatment. It is used to treat patients during pregnancy to avoid exposure of the fetus to cytotoxic drugs. The cells harvested from patients in the chronic phase of CGL can be used to treat patients with granulocytosis and severe infection (page 92).

In *acute leukaemia* a very high white count (>150 × 10⁹/l) may lead to viscosity problems and red cell transfusion for anaemia should be delayed until the white cell count has been brought down either by chemotherapy or, if indicated, by leukapheresis as this may lead to rapid clinical deterioration.

Leukapheresis has also been used for symptomatic improvement in Sézary syndrome and hairy cell leukaemia.

Plasma exchange

Plasma exchange has been used in the management of a large number of diseases, but in only a few has it proved to be of real benefit to the patient. Even in these patients it is almost always only a holding operation until other forms of treatment become effective.

Hyperviscosity syndrome

This occurs as a complication of macroglobinaemia or multiple myeloma when the amount of paraprotein is so large that it affects the plasma viscosity. The features of this include tiredness, headache, loss of appetite, haemorrhage, cardiac failure, fits, hemiplegia and clouding of consciousness. The retinal veins show irregular sausage-shaped dilatation, and there may be papilloedema. The relative viscosity is usually above 4.0. A total plasma exchange with PPF will remove about 40% of the patient's own plasma and reduce the viscosity accordingly. The plasma exchange should be repeated daily or on alternate days until relief of symptoms occurs, after which it is repeated when the patient's symptoms recur. The underlying condition should also be treated. Transfusion will raise the whole blood viscosity further and should be delayed in anaemic patients until plasma exchange has been carried out.

Renal failure occurring in multiple myeloma is usually not affected by plasma exchange, unless it is of recent onset and rapidly progressive when plasma exchange may prevent further renal deterioration and occasionally will cause some improvement.

Thrombotic thrombocytopenic purpura

This rare disorder consists of thrombocytopenia, microangiopathic haemolytic anaemia, fluctuating neurological involvement and renal failure. In this condition plasma exchange with FFP is used to halt acute progression of the disease. It may initially have to be carried out daily, and, when remission is achieved, repeated at two- to three-week intervals. Success in this condition may be due to the supply of a plasma factor mediating the release of endothelial prostacyclin. Simple infusion of FFP may be all that is necessary to maintain improvement.

In haemolytic uraemic syndrome plasmapheresis has been tried for the same reasons as in TTP but with little success.

Systemic lupus erythematosus (SLE)

In SLE plasma exchange may be useful in halting progressive disease by removing circulating and tissue bound immune complexes. Complications which have responded to plasma exchange after failure of conventional therapy are lupus nephritis, cerebral lupus and pulmonary vasculitis and serositis.

Plasma exchange has also been used in rapidly progressive nephritis, such as that due to *polyarteritis nodosa* and *Wegener's granulomatosis, myositis* and *scleroderma* with improvement in some patients, but no effect in others.

Removal of antibodies

The removal of autoantibodies by plasma exchange is useful in only a few specific instances.

Antiglomerular basement membrane antibody

These antibodies cause *Goodpasture's syndrome*, the association of rapidly progressive nephritis and pulmonary haemorrhage. Plasma exchange used early in the disease limits the degree of renal failure and prevents pulmonary haemorrhage.

Myasthenia gravis

Myasthenia gravis due to anti-acetylcholine receptor antibodies shows striking clinical improvement on plasma exchange. This begins two to three days after plasmapheresis and lasts for about the same period of time. It is used in myasthenic crisis and in the preparation of patients for thymectomy. Remission can often be maintained if plasmapheresis is followed by immunosuppression. In *Eaton-Lambert syndrome* plasma exchange seems to be of some value, but improvement is not seen until 10–20 days after the start of treatment.

Diabetes

Autoantibodies to the insulin receptor cause some cases of severe insulin resistant diabetes and these respond to plasma exchange and immuno-suppression.

In juvenile diabetes plasma exchange has been tried at presentation to remove anti-islet cell antibodies to preserve as much islet function as possible, but there is no evidence that it is of benefit.

Antibodies to coagulation factors

Plasma exchange lowers the amount of these antibodies in the blood and is useful in cases where there is an urgent need for replacement therapy, for example preparation for surgery, to reduce the dose of coagulation factor needed to achieve haemostasis.

Autoimmune haemolytic anaemia (AIHA)

Plasma exchange has been tried in both cold agglutinin disease and warm AIHA in very severely affected patients unresponsive to conventional therapy, but is usually ineffective because most of the antibody is bound to the red cells. In cold agglutinin disease there is also great difficulty in preventing agglutination of the cells while out of the body. A more logical approach is whole blood exchange and in some patients this has been useful.

Immune thrombocytopenic purpura

In this condition immune suppression, splenectomy and treatment with high dose γ-globulin (page 119) are usually used, but in rare unresponsive patients plasmapheresis has been tried with success in some cases.

Anticardiolipin antibodies

There is an association between high titre anticardiolipin antibodies and the lupus anticoagulant with spontaneous abortions and thrombocytopenia. Trials are under way to treat women with the antibody and a history of repeated abortions by repeated plasma exchange as an adjunct to treatment with steroids.

Cryoglobulinaemia

Cryoglobulinaemia is due to the occurrence of antibodies which will precipitate reversibly in the cold, associated with lymphoproliferative disorders, autoimmune and infectious disorders. In severe cases plasma exchange is useful to relieve symptoms until treatment of the underlying disease takes effect. In this condition the patient's own plasma can be used for plasma exchange. The plasma collected at the first exchange is kept at 4°C until needed, when the cryoprecipitate is spun off and the cryoglobulin free plasma used.

Removal of other antibodies

Haemolytic disease of the newborn (page 158), post-transfusion purpura (page 32) and in BMT with an ABO incompatible donor (page

171) have already been discussed. Removal of alloantibodies to high frequency blood group antigens may allow transfusion when the required blood cannot be obtained. In aplastic anaemia due to antibodies plasma exchange has been tried with occasional success in pure red cell aplasia.

Miscellaneous conditions

Removal of protein bound poisons in thyroxine overdose, mushroom poisoning (charcoal perfusion of separated plasma can also be used), and methyl parathion poisoning can only be achieved by PE.

In the inherited inability to α-oxidize phytanic acid, *Refsum's disease*, phytanic acid collects in the tissues. This causes polyneuropathy, retinitis and eventually death. This can be prevented by a chlorophyl free diet. Plasma exchange gradually removes any phytanic acid which has already accumulated in the tissues.

In homozygotes with *inherited hyperlipidaemia* long-term plasma exchange carried out fortnightly results in slower progression of this fatal disease.

In Guillain-Barré syndrome and related disorders variable results have been reported anecdotally and trials have given discordant results. At present plasma exchange is reserved for acute, severe cases.

Plasma exchange has also been tried in a number of other conditions. In some, pemphigus, rheumatoid arthritis, multiple sclerosis, and renal graft rejection, variable results with many failures have been reported. In psoriasis, Raynaud's phenomenon and Fabry's disease, there was no effect. In all these conditions it is probably of no use.

Further reading

Tindall, R S A (Ed.) (1982) Therapeutic apheresis and perfusion. Alan R Liss, Inc., New York.

Taft, E G (1983) Therapeutic apheresis. *Human Pathology*, 14, 235.

Urbaniak, S J (1984) Therapeutic plasma and cellular apheresis. *Clinics in Haematology*, 13, 217.

Westphal, R G (1984) Health risks to cytapheresis donors. *Clinics in Haematology*, 13, 289.

13 Plasma and red cell substitutes

Non-human colloids

Albumin-containing solutions are expensive to prepare and human plasma is a limited resource. They are difficult to transport and store and may carry a hepatitis and AIDS risk. These factors have stimulated research into non-human colloids for use as blood volume expanders capable of providing an oncotic effect.

Because of their synthetic nature these products have side effects, some of which can be exploited therapeutically. A description of the commonly used synthetic colloids and their use follows.

Dextrans

Dextrans are high molecular weight polysaccharides, produced by the action of a bacterial enzyme, dextran-sucrase, when leuconostoc bacteria are grown in a sucrose-containing medium. Depending on the strain of bacterium used and other modifications the exact structure of the molecule produced varies. In general the predominant linkage between glucose residues is the α-1,6-glucosidic linkage. The molecules therefore have a low degree of branching. Different molecular sizes are subsequently obtained by acid hydrolysis. The dextrans are fractionated, according to molecular weight. The two most commonly used preparations are dextran 40 (average mol. wt 40,000) and dextran 70 (average mol. wt 70,000). They are provided in solution in 0.9% saline or 5% glucose (Table 13.1). They can be stored at room temperature for up to ten years.

Properties of dextrans in vivo

After infusion the half-life of dextran depends on its molecular size

Table 13.1 The properties of synthetic volume expanders

Product	Availability	MW (Daltons)	Plasma $t_{\frac{1}{2}}$ (hours)	Maximum dose	Notes
Dextran 40	10% in saline or dextrose	15–75,000	4	1st day 2 g/kg/24 h then 1 g/kg/24 h	Has antithrombin effect and improves capillary perfusion
Dextran 70	6% in saline or dextrose	20–115,000	15	1st day 1.2 g/kg/24 h then 0.6 g/kg/24 h	Volume expansion
Pectin Hydroxyethyl starch HES (450/0.7)	6% in saline	40–100,000	12	1,500 ml/24 h	Red cell sedimenting agent, volume expansion
Gelatin Haemaccel (urea bridged) Plamagel (modified fluid)	3.5% in electrolyte solution	25–35,000 30–40,000	4		Volume expansion, plasma exchange, N.B. cannot be added to citrated blood due to Ca^{++} content

distribution. Smaller molecules are rapidly lost. Dextran 70 has a half-life of around ten hours, that of dextran 40 is four hours.

Because of its smaller molecular weight dextran 40 has a greater oncotic effect and blood volume expanding effect immediately after infusion than dextran 70. With dextran 40 the blood volume expansion effect has been lost by six hours, whereas 30% of the volume expansion achieved by dextran 70 is still present at 24 hours. In practice dextran 40 and dextran 70 have a water retaining effect of approximately 20–25 ml/g within the circulation.

The bulk of infused dextran is excreted unchanged in the urine, the renal threshold being at a molecular weight of around 50,000 in normal individuals. The remaining dextran is taken up by liver, spleen, kidneys, brain and muscle and broken down to carbon dioxide and water.

Use of dextrans in clinical practice

VOLUME REPLACEMENT

Dextran 40 and dextran 70 can both be used as volume replacement fluids during acute blood loss; they improve blood pressure, increase cardiac output and reduce peripheral resistance. Dextran 40 is said to have a more beneficial effect on tissue oxygenation by improving capillary perfusion.

Colloids for volume replacement should be given in electrolyte solution rather than dextrose. Because they appear in the urine these molecules have an osmotic diuretic effect. This is greatest with dextran 40, which should therefore be avoided in patients with initial haemoconcentration.

In general, dextran 70 is preferable to dextran 40 as a volume replacement fluid, its effect being better sustained. Five hundred to one thousand millilitres can be infused initially, further infusion being guided by CVP measurements. In acute, severe haemorrhage the aim is to prevent the haematocrit falling below 30%. In a patient without pre-existing anaemia this means a maximum volume of 1,500 ml can be infused, thereafter blood transfusion will be needed. (See page 57 for treatment of acute blood loss).

USE OF DEXTRANS IN THROMBOTIC STATES

Dextrans have an antithrombotic effect, causing dilution of the coagulation factors. They also adhere to platelet surfaces stabilizing them and interfering with the interaction between platelets, factor VIII related antigen and the blood vessel wall. Clots formed in the presence of dextrans are more friable than normal, the fibrin molecule being less strong. Most macromolecules used in volume expansion solutions have similar effects, but to a lesser degree than dextrans. These effects on coagulation are not important in the previously normal individual until over 1–1.5 g/kg body weight has been given. Obviously synthetic colloids should be avoided in the thrombocytopenic and those with coagulation defects.

These effects on coagulation have been exploited in the prophylaxis of thromboembolism. An infusion of 100 ml dextran 70 in six hours prior to and over the time of major surgery has been shown to reduce the incidence of subsequent fatal pulmonary embolism. Dextran 40 has also been used during vascular surgery.

ISCHAEMIC CONDITIONS

Dextrans 70 and 40 can be used to improve tissue perfusion in ischaemic conditions such as embolism, diabetic gangrene and scleroderma.

OTHER USES OF DEXTRANS

Macromolecules such as dextran within the plasma act like capacitors, reducing the electric repulsion normally existing between cells (zeta potential) causing rouleaux formation. This is exploited to cause more rapid and efficient sedimentation of red cells during harvesting of platelets and/or white cells from single donors by cell separators (page 180). Dextran 40, 5% in electrolyte solution is also used to wash out blood from cadaver organs to be used for transplantation.

Hazards of dextran infusion

Dextrans have similar effects to those of albumin but lack its transport function. They are thus useful in blood volume replacement where hypoproteinaemia is not a factor.

ALLERGIC HAZARDS

Because dextrans occur naturally, many individuals possess dextran antibodies and allergic reactions such as fever, flushing and tachycardia are common; rarely anaphylaxis may occur. However, the occurrence of allergic reactions is less common than with human products. Non-immune reactions may occur due to the release of histamines triggered by the rapid infusion of macromolecules.

RENAL TOXICITY

Dextrans with molecular weights below 60,000 are filtered by the glomerulus; if they become concentrated they may block the renal tubule. They may also accumulate in the cells of the proximal tubule. Dextrans may therefore cause acute renal failure. This is more likely if they are given at rates exceeding one litre daily, or when the blood urea is over 10 mmol/l (60 mg/100 ml) or if the urine output is under 1,500 ml per day. When it is proposed to use dextrans electively to improve tissue perfusion these factors must be taken into account. In the acute situation if renal status is uncertain it is best to avoid the use of dextrans.

HAEMOSTATIC DEFECTS

Primary haemostatis (a function of platelet/vessel wall interaction) and clot stability are compromised by macromolecules, but in practice these effects are not hazardous provided less than 1–1.5 g/kg body weight dextran is infused.

RED-CELL PSEUDOAGGLUTINATION

Rouleaux formation may give the appearance of agglutinates (i.e. false positives) during blood grouping tests. It is recommended that blood for cross-matching be withdrawn before the infusion. However, at the doses normally used this is not a common problem. Should pseudo-agglutinates occur, they can be distinguished from true agglutinates by the fact that they will disperse on addition of normal saline.

Hydroxyethyl starch

Maize or sorghum starch consists predominantly of amylopectin, a highly branched polysaccharide similar to glycogen. Chemical modification of this by ethylene oxide produces hydroxyethyl starch (HES). Molecules of various sizes can be made, and these may contain variable numbers of substituted hydroxyethyl groups. The product is therefore defined by its molecular weight and the degree of hydroxyethyl group substitution. The latter affects the metabolism of the molecule *in vivo*.

Two preparations are in common use: HES 450/0.70 (mol. wt 450,000, degree of substitution 70%) and HES 264/0.43.

Properties of HES in vivo

Immediately after infusion HES 264/0.43, being a relatively small molecule, is a potent oncotic agent, but relatively little is present after 24 hours, so its effects are short-lived. The short half-life is not simply due to urinary loss but also to rapid metabolism by plasma alpha amylase. This preparation is not generally available.

HES 450/0.70 is a much larger molecule and, because it is highly substituted (70%), it is more resistant to the action of amylase. Thus it is retained for long periods in the plasma, and its effects are similar to those of dextran 70.

The clinical uses of HES are similar to those of dextrans. However, it is not yet licensed for use as a volume expander in the UK, and is mostly used as a red cell sedimenting agent in cell separation (pages 180). Its effect on primary haemostasis is less marked than dextran and it is not used as an antithrombotic agent. With large doses (greater than 2 litres per day) multiple coagulation defects can occur. The effect of HES is prolonged in patients with renal failure. It does not appear to cause histamine release.

HES also causes infrequent anaphylactic reactions. Vomiting, fever, chills and itching have been reported. The latter symptoms may last for a week or more as HES is only slowly lost from the body.

Modified gelatine

Therapeutic colloids are derived from cattle bone gelatine by various methods. Modified fluid gelatin (e.g. Plasmagel, Plasmion) and urea-bridged gelatin (Haemaccel), have molecular weights of around 35,000. Haemaccel is a commonly used preparation which is provided in a 3.8% solution in electrolyte solution containing Na^+ 145, Cl^- 145, K^+ 5.1 and Ca^{++} 6.25 mmol/litre (Table 13.1). Water retention capacity is around 38 ml per gram of colloid.

Properties in vivo

Gelatins are difficult to identify and isolate once infused, so little is known about their metabolism. The half-life is from four to eight hours. Seventy to ninety per cent of the molecules are below the renal threshold and therefore rapidly eliminated in the urine. Their use can be followed by a marked osmotic diuresis, and adequate fluid replacement must be provided during this phase.

Some gelatin preparations have a high calcium content and should not be given at the same time as blood. They may also be dangerous in patients with cardiac dysfunction, particularly those on digitalis.

Uses and side effects of gelatin-based colloids are comparable with those of other macromolecules. But they are mainly used in plasma exchange. Again they are not used as antithrombotic agents.

Red cell substitutes

Red cell containing preparations are expensive to prepare and store, and inconvenient to transport. Their use involves the risk of immunological transfusion reactions and infections such as hepatitis B. These problems have stimulated the search for substitutes which might provide oxygen transport function.

Cell free haemoglobin

The most obvious red cell substitute is cell free haemoglobin, which could be obtained from time-expired blood. It is now possible to crystallize haemoglobin after which multiple washing leaves a product free of cell stroma, which is not nephrotoxic. This product can be freeze dried and stored for 12 months at 4°C, or 6 months at room temperature without deterioration.

Unfortunately when reconstituted and infused these solutions consist mainly of dimeric haemoglobin which have such a high oxygen affinity that they are not useful for the delivery of oxygen to the tissues. Following infusion these molecules are bound to plasma haptoglobin until the capacity of the latter is exceeded (50–150 mg Hb/dl). The haptoglobin–haemoglobin complex is removed by the reticuloendothelial system.

As larger amounts are infused, free haemoglobin is taken up directly by the liver or lost in the urine. Thus the half-life of infused stroma-free haemoglobin is between one and seven hours. This means that the oxygen-carrying and oncotic properties of the infused haemoglobin are rapidly lost and repeated doses would be necessary. When the plasma concentration exceeds 7 g/dl the oncotic effect is considerable. The appearance of an osmotically active molecule in the urine also results in an osmotic diuresis and volume depletion. This would be exactly the opposite of the desired effect when treating active bleeding.

Methods of cross-linking haemoglobin molecules have been explored. In general, although they improve vascular retention, they increase the oxygen affinity of the molecule and thus reduce oxygen availability to the tissues. Combining haemoglobin with pyridoxal 5-phosphate improves the vascular retention of the molecule while maintaining near normal oxygen affinity, and this compound may become a useful blood substitute.

Haemoglobin can also be encapsulated in liposomes to produce artificial red cells. To produce sufficiently long-lived 'haemosomes' with a normal oxygen dissociation curve needs the development of liposomes with increased stability and the right haemoglobin derivatives, for example, reaction with pyridoxal-5-phosphate to bring the oxygen affinity into the physiological range. Such haemosomes could be freeze died for prolonged storage and reconstituted for use.

To date, clinical experience with haemoglobin solutions, cross-linked or modified haemoglobins, or liposomes is limited.

Perfluorocarbons as red cell substitutes

Perfluorocarbons are stable, biologically inert compounds consisting of ring or chain form hydrocarbons fully substituted with fluorine. Because some of them, in liquid state, can dissolve oxygen and carbon dioxide reversibly their use as blood substitutes has been explored. In order to obtain a product suitable for infusion the perfluorocarbon must be emulsified to a suitable particle size ($<0.1\,\mu m$) which is non-toxic and of acceptable viscosity. An oncotic agent such as hydroxyethyl starch (HES) must also be added.

The commercial preparation Fluosol DA (20%) (*Green Cross Corporation Osaka, Japan*) contains the fluorocarbons perfluorotripropylamine and perfluorodecalin. The emulsifier is Pluoronic F-68 and the oncotic agent HES.

Following infusion the half-life is around 13 hours and the tissue retention time, largely due to F-tripropylamine, is 65 days. The perfluorocarbons are taken up by the reticuloendothelial system and eventually excreted via the lungs. The emulsifier is excreted unchanged in the urine and faeces, while the HES is metabolized.

Oxygen and carbon dioxide uptake and release by perfluorocarbon solutions occur at about twice the rate achieved by human haemoglobin solutions. Unfortunately the capacity to dissolve gases is compromised by emulsification, so that the patient must breathe oxygen enriched air in order that sufficient oxygen is dissolved by the perfluorocarbon *in vivo*. At least 60% oxygen in inspired air is required. A 20% solution would give about 60% of the oxygen delivery to the tissues achieved by normal blood.

Fluosol DA has a low toxicity. Very few anaphylactic reactions have been encountered. There have been no significant disturbances of co-agulation function or bleeding time during its use. Transient increases in the liver enzyme SGOT have been observed. Rarely, patients may develop pulmonary reactions with dyspnoea and pulmonary hypertension. This is thought to be due to the activation of complement by the Pluronic F68 emulsifier. Steroids may prevent this.

Fluosol DA has been given as an initial infusion of 20 ml/kg body weight, followed by doses of 10 ml/kg after 12 hours, if necessary. It is infused at rates not exceeding 10 ml/minute. Besides the oxygen delivery effect Fluosol DA has a marked plasma expansive effect. The compound has been used in surgery in patients who have refused blood transfusions on religious grounds or when blood was not available. It has also been used as a plasma expander in burns, in coronary angiography and as a cold perfusate for cadaver organs for transplantation.

In future these low viscosity gas transport emulsions may be found superior to red cells for certain indications, reaching parts red cells fail to reach in, for example, ischaemic vascular conditions. They may also transport oxygen to areas of anerobic infection helping to limit and cure these.

Further reading

Hulse, J D, Yakobi, A (1983) Hetastarch: an overview of the colloid and its metabolism. *Drug Intelligence and Clinical Pharmacy*, **17**, 334.

Ross, A D, Angaran, D M (1984) Colloids *vs*. crystalloids—a continuing controversy. *Drug Intelligence and Clinical Pharmacy*, **18**, 202.

Mishler IV, J M (1984) Synthetic plasma expanders—their pharmacology, safety and clinical efficacy. *Clinics in Haematoogy*, **18**, 75.

Wickham, N W R, Hardy, R N (1982) Artificial blood from fluorocarbons. *Hospital Update*, **12**, 1433.

Gruber, U F (1969) *Blood Replacement*. Springer Verlag, Heidelberg.

Rudowski, W J (1980) Evaluation of modern plasma expanders and blood substitutes. *British Journal of Hospital Medicine*, April, 389–398.

De Venuto (1979) Appraisal of haemoglobin solution as a blood substitute. *Surgery Gynaecology and Obstetrics*, **149**, 417–436.

14 Principles of blood transfusion serology

Factors affecting blood group antibody/antigen reactions

Antibody related factors

The affinity of the antibody for the antigen

In general, the antibody first produced after primary antigenic challenge has relatively poorer affinity for its antigen than antibody produced later. This is true for both IgM and IgG antibodies. The greater the affinity or 'fit' between antibody and antigen the stronger the reaction between them. There are no technical manipulations that can alter this phenomenon, but it has to be taken into account in serological testing. For example, when screening serum for antibody a panel of red cells, which are homozygous for all the important red cell antigens, will ensure detection of any weak antibodies present. Similarly during red cell grouping, the specific antisera used must be able to agglutinate control red cells heterozygous for their antigen.

The class of antibody

Immediately after primary challenge with most blood group antigens such as rhesus system antigens, IgM is produced. Later in the response and also after a secondary challenge, IgG predominates. Unless challenge with non-self antigen on red cells during transfusion or pregnancy has occurred, no antibody is present.

However, the ABO system is different because from shortly after birth the appropriate non-self ABO antibody is present (page 10). This is almost always IgM. This is probably due to the fortuitous presence of ABO-like antigens on bacteria. Since these antigens are polysaccharides with simple repeating antigenic groups, they act as T lymphocyte independent antigens. Such antigens activate appropriate clones of B2 lymphocytes directly and result in the production of IgM antibodies. Only individuals of group O readily produce ABO IgG 'immune' antibodies.

IgM is at least pentavalent, having ten antibody combining sites (page 124). This property and its large molecular size mean that IgM can easily bridge the gap that normally exists between red cells due to their mutual repulsion. IgM antibody, therefore, readily causes agglutination in saline; this reaction is strongest at 4°C. Hence these antibodies are frequently described as 'saline' or 'cold' agglutinins.

IgG molecules have only two antigen combining sites and are smaller. They react best with the appropriate antigen at 37°C. Although they readily coat the red cells, they often fail to bridge the gap between adjacent cells to produce agglutination. Several laboratory techniques are available which facilitate agglutination of IgG coated red cells and allow detection of such antibody–antigen reactions. The most important of these is the antiglobulin (Coombs') test. The reaction of various antibodies in serological tests are given in Table 14.1 and their clinical significance is outlined in Table 14.2.

Antigen related factors

The size and distribution of antigen

Blood group antigens of large molecular size, projecting from the red cell membrane are more accessible to the corresponding antibody. If they are densely distributed, or mobile within the membrane, then it is more likely that following reaction with antibody, the Fc portions of the latter will interact with and fix complement. ABO antigens have these properties, rhesus antigens lack them.

The distance between red cells

Red cells have a negative surface charge due to the carboxyl groups present on the sialic acid side chains and therefore repel each other. The gap between the red cells caused by this 'ζ' potential is easily bridged by IgM antibodies. IgG antibodies coat the red cells but fail to cause agglutination. A number of techniques are used to reduce the distance between adjacent red cells and facilitate agglutination by IgG antibodies.

Table 14.1   Characteristics of blood group antibodies (*Courtesy of Ortho Diagnostic Systems*)

Antibody	Saline	Albumin	AHG	Enzyme	Optimum temp °C	Invitro haemoly-sis	% Blood compat-ible
ABO system							
Anti-A	Yes	Yes	Some	Yes	4-20	Yes	55
Anti-A$_1$	Yes	No	No		4	No	64
Anti-B	Yes	Yes	Some	Yes	4-20	Yes	88
Anti-A,B	Yes	Yes	Some		4-20	Yes	44
Anti-H	Yes	Some	Some		4	Yes	0
Rhesus system							
Anti-D	Some	Yes	Yes	Yes	37	No	15
Anti-C	Some	Yes	Yes	Yes	37	No	30
Anti-E	Yes	Yes	Yes	Yes	37	No	70
Anti-c	Some	Yes	Yes	Yes	37	No	20
Anti-e	Some	Yes	Yes	Yes	37	No	3
Anti-f	Some	Yes	Yes	Yes	37	No	33
Anti-C^w	Yes	Yes	Yes	Yes	37	No	98
Anti-G	Rare	Yes	Yes	Yes	37	No	15
Anti-V	Rare	Rare	Yes	Yes	37	No	100C 82N

Antibody	Saline	Albumin	AHG	Enzyme	Optimum temp °C	Invitro haemoly-sis	% Blood compat-ible
Kell system							
Anti-K	Some	Some	Yes	Some	37	No	90C 97N
Anti-k	Rare	Rare	Yes		37	No	0.2C <0.1N
Anti-Kp^a	Rare	Rare	Yes		37	No	98C >99N
Anti-Kp^b	Rare	Rare	Yes		37	No	<0.1C <0.1N
Anti-Js^a	Rare	Rare	Yes		37	No	>99C 80N
Anti-Js^b	Rare	Rare	Yes	Some	37	No	0C <0.1N
Duffy system							
Anti-Fy^a	Rare	Rare	Yes	No	37	No	33C 89N
Anti-Fy^b	Rare	Rare	Yes	No	37	No	20C 77N
Kidd system							
Anti-Jk^a	Rare	Rare	Yes	Yes	37	No	25C 9N
Anti-Jk^b	Rare	Rare	Yes	Yes	37	No	25C
Anti-Jk^{ab}	No	No	Yes	Yes	37		0

C-Caucasian N-Negro M-Male F-Female

Antibody	Saline	Albumin	AHG	Enzyme	Optimum temp °C	In vitro haemolysis	% Blood compatible
Lewis system							
Anti-Le^a	Yes	Yes	Yes	Yes	5-37	Some	78C 82N
Anti-Le^b	Yes	Yes	Yes	Yes	5-37	Some	28C 40N
MNS system							
Anti-M	Yes	Yes	Some	No	5-25	No	22C 63N
Anti-N	Yes	Yes	Rare	No	5-25	No	28C 39N
Anti-S	Some	Some	Yes	No	25-37	No	45
Anti-s	Rare	Rare	Yes	Yes	37	Yes	11
Anti-U	Rare	Rare	Yes	Yes	37	Yes	0C <1N
P system							
Anti-P$_1$	Yes	Yes	Some	Some	5-25	No	21C 5N
Anti-P	Yes	Yes	Yes		5-37	Yes	<0.1
Anti-P+P$_1$ +P^k (Tja)	Yes	Yes	Yes		5-37	Yes	<0.1
I system							
Anti-I	Yes	Yes	Rare	Yes	5-25	No	<0.1
Anti-i	Yes	Yes	Rare	Yes	5-25	No	>99

Antibody	Saline	Albumin	AHG	Enzyme	Optimum temp °C	Invitro haemolysis	% Blood compatible
Lutheran system							
Anti-Lu[a]	Yes	Yes	Rare		25	No	92
Anti-Lu[b]	Rare	Rare	Yes	Yes	37	No	<1.0
Other systems							
Anti-Bi[a] (Biles)	Rare	Rare	Yes		37	No	>99
Anti-Yt[a] (Cartwright)	Rare	Rare	Yes		37	No	<0.1
Anti-Ch[a] (Chido)	Rare	Rare	Yes		37	No	1.7
Anti-Cs[a] (Cost-Sterling)	Rare	Rare	Yes		37	No	2
Anti-Di[a] (Diego)	Rare	Rare	Yes		37	No	>99
Anti-Ge (Gerbich)	Some	Some	Yes		25–37	No	<0.1
Anti-Sc:2 (Scianna)	Rare	Rare	Yes		37	No	>99
Anti-Vel	Some	Some	Yes	Some	37	Some	<1.0
Anti-Wr[a] (Wright)	Yes	Yes	Yes		25-37	No	>99
Anti-Yk[a] (York)	Rare	Rare	Yes		37	No	5
Anti-Xg[a]	Rare	Rare	Yes		37	No	36♂ 13♀

Table 14.2 Blood group antibodies and their clinical significance

GROUP antibody	Occurrence	Haemolytic disease of the newborn HDN	Haemolytic transfusion reactions HTR	Notes
ABO	Common	Yes	Yes	See page 10, Table 2.3, HDN page 161.
LEWIS				
anti-Le^a	<0.5%	No	V. rare, M ⟶ s*	Most react in the cold; haemolysis mainly extravascular. Lewis antigens not developed in the fetus. Lewis antibodies may cause graft rejection.
anti-Le^b	Rare and weak	No	V. rare, M ⟶ s	
P				
anti-P₁	Table 2.5	No	V. v. rare	The Donath Landsteiner antibody has anti-P specificity (page 224).
Ii				
anti-I	Common	No	Yes	Common as autoantibodies
anti-i				
RHESUS				These are immune antibodies, mainly IgG but IgM and IgA also found. Anti-C, anti-E and anti-G mainly found with anti-D.
anti-D				
anti-C				
anti-E		M ⟶ S	M ⟶ S	
anti-G				Anti-E may be naturally occurring.
anti-C^w				Anti-C^w can be found in C and c individuals.
anti-c				Anti-CD, anti-CE, anti-CDE, anti-ce and anti-Ce occur and can cause HDN or HTR.
anti-e				

	Frequency	Severity*	Severity*	
KELL				
anti-K	Rare	M → S	M → S	KK genotype only 1:500
anti-k	V. rare	M → S	M → S	

Other Kell antibodies, anti-Kp^a, anti-Kp^b, anti-Js^a and anti-Js^b occur very rarely and can cause HDN or HTR. Anti-KL occurs after transfusion in Mcleod's syndrome.

	Frequency	Severity*	Severity*	
DUFFY				
anti-Fy^a	V. rare	M → S	M → S	
anti-Fy^b	V. v. rare	M → ?	?	
KIDD				
anti-Jk^a	Rare	M → S	M → S	These antibodies can cause delayed transfusion reactions.
anti-Jk^b	V. rare	M	M → S	
anti-Jk (a + b)	V. v. rare	M	M	Found in Fy (a−b−) individuals (page 20).
MNSs				
anti-M	V. rare	M → S	M	Other rare antibodies, anti-Mi^a, anti-Mt and anti-Vw have caused HDN and HTR.
anti-N	V. rare	M	M	
anti-S	Rare	M → S	M → S	Anti-Nf is found in renal dialysis patients.
anti-s	V. rare	M → S	M → S	
anti-U	More common in Blacks	M → S	I → S	
LUTHERAN				
anti-Lu^a	Rare	M	M	Delayed transfusion reactions.
anti-Lu^b	Rare	M	M	

Other antibodies which have very rarely caused HDN or HTR include: anti-Do; anti-Di^a, anti-Di^b; anti-Wr^a; anti-Co; anti-Ye^a; anti-Ge; anti-At^a; anti-Lan; anti-Jr^a and anti-En^a. There are also some extremely rare (private) antigens and antibodies against these can cause HDN (page 155), but are highly unlikely to cause HTR.

* Indicates severity: M = mild, I = intermediate and S = severe

Addition of albumin

Bovine serum albumin (1–2 drops of a 20% solution) is often added to the incubation mixture. The colloid molecules are thought to act as capacitors reducing the charge between the red cells and bringing them closer together. The disadvantages to its use are expense and the tendency for the cells to become sticky and form rouleaux, which may be misinterpreted as agglutinates.

Enzyme treatment of red cells

Enzymes such as papain, ficin, bromelin or trypsin cleave some of the proteins off the red cell membrane, coincidentally removing some sugar residues and reducing the negative surface charge. The red cells may be pretreated with the enzyme, or it may be added directly to the reaction mixture. This procedure increases the sensitivity of some antigen/antibody reactions particularly of the rhesus system. Unfortunately other antigens are destroyed by enzyme treatment (Table 14.3).

Table 14.3   Effect of enzyme treatment on various red cell antigens

Antigens weakened	Antibody/antigen reaction strengthened
Duffy, MNSs	All rhesus groups
En^a, Lu^a, Yt^a	Le^a, Le^b
Xg^a, Ge, Ch, Rg	P$_1$, Jk^a (IAT),
Tn, Pr,	I, i
T (high enzyme conc.)	

Use of Low Ionic Strength Saline (LISS)

When normal saline is used the Na$^+$ and Cl$^-$ ions interact with negatively and postively charged groups respectively on the antigen and antibody reducing their interaction. The use of LISS (0.2 M NaCl in 7% glycine) speeds red cell antigen antibody interaction and is also more sensitive. This allows rapid cross-matching and antibody detection, but occasionally causes non-specific adsorption of antibody on to red cells. It may not detect antibodies to the Kell system antigens as well as they are detected by other techniques. Many laboratories use LISS in most of their serology tests.

There are also modifications to the LISS technique, such as the addition of protamine (LIP) or polybrene (LISP), but these are more complicated and are not generally used. The addition of polybrene is very sensitive for the detection of rhesus interactions, but is less sensitive for the Kell system.

Centrifugation

Using any of the above methods the reaction between cells may be enhanced by low speed centrifugation (1,000 rpm) of the reaction mixture. This allows reduction of the incubation time. However, care is required as false agglutination may result from too long or too fast centrifugation.

The antiglobulin or Coombs' test

The antiglobulin test detects antibody coating of the red cells and is used to detect antibodies such as IgG which react with red cells without causing agglutination.

In the test the antibody coated red cells are reacted with a second antibody directed against the antibody already on the cells. This second antibody, anti-human globulin or AHG, usually produced in rabbits, cross-links the antibody on different cells producing agglutination (Fig. 14.1). There are two versions of the test:

1 The direct antiglobulin test (DAT) in which the coating of the red cells has taken place in the body before the blood is taken.
2 The indirect antiglobulin test (IAT) in which the coating of the red cells with the first antibody is carried out *in vitro*.

The direct antiglobulin test is used to detect specific antibody reaction with the red cells which has occurred *in vivo* in autoimmune haemolytic anaemia or haemolytic disease of the newborn. The red cells are washed to remove *all* traces of unattached antibodies and are then incubated with the rabbit AHG. This reacts with any antibody adhering to the red cells and causes visible agglutination by linking the antibody coated cells. It is very important that the cells are well washed, if any free γ-globulin from the serum is allowed to remain, it would react with the AHG, preventing its attachment to the red cell bound immunoglobulin. Thus the addition of AHG would fail to agglutinate sensitized cells producing a false negative result.

In the indirect antiglobulin test the initial coating of the red cells is done by incubating the red cells with serum at 37°C. The red cells are then washed and AHG is added as above. If coating has taken

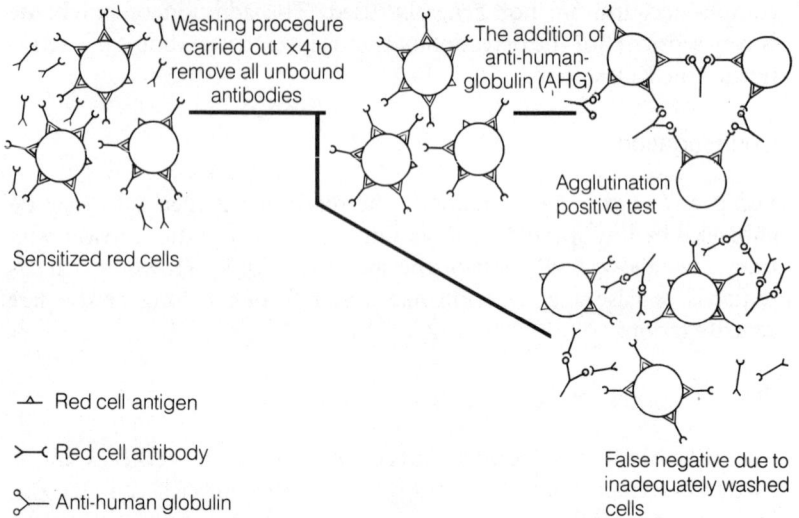

— Red cell antigen

— Red cell antibody

— Anti-human globulin

Fig. 14.1   The antiglobulin test (Coombs' test). In the direct test the cells are sensitized in vivo; in the indirect test the cells are sensitized in vitro.

place, agglutination will occur. The indirect test is used in three different ways in serology:

1   to detect antibodies in serum,
2   to detect antigens on red cells—blood grouping,
3   to detect antigen/antibody pairs in donor red cell/recipient serum mixtures—cross-matching.

Anti-human globulin for routine use in blood banks is usually 'broad spectrum' AHG and contains rabbit anti-human-IgG and anti-human-complement. However, by immunizing rabbits with purified antigens, specific anti-human-IgG, -IgM, -IgA -C_3, C_4, etc. can be made. These may yield useful information when investigating autoimmune haemolysis or drug induced haemolysis.

IgG antibodies can be converted to give saline reaction by treatment with dithiothereotol (DTT). This acts by reducing some disulphide bridges, which, when the DTT is dialysed out, reform randomly forming aggregated IgG resembling IgM.

Securing safe blood for transfusion

In order to avoid serious blood transfusion reactions several conditions must be met:

1 Donor and recipient must be ABO compatible because antibodies for this system occur 'naturally'.

2 Donor and recipient must be Rh (D) identical because although anti-D does not occur naturally it forms readily in response to transfusion or transplacental bleeding. Fifteen per cent of the population are D-negative and the consequences of sensitization are serious (page 121).

3 The serum of the recipient should not contain any antibody reactive against the donor red cell antigens.

4 The donor plasma should not contain high titre ABO antibodies. Other blood group antibodies are less dangerous as they are sufficiently diluted in the recipient's plasma.

5 The presence of an autoantibody in the recipient should be excluded as this makes the interpretation of grouping and cross-matching results difficult.

Conditions 1 and 2 are satisfied by ABO and Rh (D) grouping. Rhesus negative (dd) donors are fully rhesus genotyped, only cde/cde blood being labelled Rh negative (but see page 14). D-negative recipients are only genotyped if previous haemolytic transfusion reactions or haemolytic disease of the newborn have occurred.

Condition 3 is met by cross-matching recipient serum against donor red cells, in addition the recipient's serum is often screened for antibody against a panel of red cells of known antigenicity.

Condition 4 is met by identifying all group O donors with anti-A or -B haemolysins at the collecting laboratory. Such blood is used for group O recipients only. Other blood group antibodies are also screened for in donor plasma, and it is particularly important to screen Rh negative donors for anti-D as their blood could be given to a neonate with haemolytic disease of the newborn.

Condition 5 is met by carrying out a direct antiglobulin test on the recipient's cells as this will exclude the presence of significant autoantibody. Alternatively, recipient serum and cells may be incubated together as an 'autologous control' during antibody screening.

Selection of blood

When a patient is to be transfused, donor units of identical ABO and Rh (D) groups are selected if available. However, individuals of groups A, B and AB may also be given group O blood. Group AB patients may also be given group A blood since B is a relatively weak antigen on AB cells. This would only be done if there were a very urgent need. Patients of subgroup A$_2$ with anti-A$_1$, inactive at 37°C can be given group A blood safely.

Premenopausal Rh negative (dd) females must never receive D-positive blood or blood products except in dire emergencies. Rh negative males who have not previously been sensitized may be given Rh positive blood if Rh negative blood cannot be supplied.

Occasionally the recipient has an antibody to a blood group antigen carried by most of the population such as 'k' (Cellano). Donors negative for such antigens are difficult to find, and many blood banks keep a register of donors negative for such groups and/or keep frozen stocks of their red cells.

Having obtained group compatible donor blood the recipient's serum is screened for the presence of significant antibodies and 'cross-matched' against the donor's red cells.

Theoretical aspects of blood transfusion serology

Blood grouping

To assign ABO groups the individual's red cells are incubated with known anti-A, anti-B and group O serum. Group O serum is included because it contains potent anti-A which will identify weak subgroups of A. Known control group A, B and O red cells are always included to ensure that the standard antisera are active, and that false positives (for example with group O cells) do not occur.

The person's (patient's) serum is also incubated with the standard cells so that the presence of the corresponding natural antibody can be confirmed. The pattern of antigens and antibodies in the ABO system is shown in Table 2.3. If there is any discrepancy, the tests should be repeated. In persons of group A$_2$ and A$_2$B the presence of anti-A$_1$ in the serum leads to anomalous results. For example, an individual of group A$_2$B may be positive on testing against anti-A and anti-B, yet have anti-A activity in serum. To confirm the presence of the A$_2$ antigen on the red cells, and anti-A$_1$ in the serum, such individuals require further testing. Known anti-A$_1$ serum, produced by adsorbing group B serum with group A$_2$ cells, is mixed with the cells of the subject under investigation and known group A cells. There should be no reaction with the subject's cells if she is group A$_2$, but the control group A$_1$ cells will be positive. The subject's serum will be active against group A cells, but not group A_2 cells. The lectin *Dolichus biflorus* reacts specifically with group A_1 cells and does not agglutinate A_2 cells. The lectin *Ulex europeus* (anti-H lectin) will give a strong reaction with A_2 cells and a weak or negative reaction with A_1 cells. These reactions are used for subtyping group A cells. Occasionally discrepancies result from abnormalities in the patient. Neonates and immune-deficient individuals have low immunoglobulins and may lack the expected ABO system antibody. Individuals of group A with carcinoma of the bowel may acquire pseudo B antigen, and may appear to be of group AB and yet possess anti-B in their serum.

D typing should be done using at least two known anti-D sera, usually one causing agglutination in saline only, 'saline anti-D', and a second requiring albumin or enzyme addition or the use of the IAT. To check for the presence of the weak form of D, Du, an antibody known to be capable of detecting it is used by the indirect antiglobulin test (IAT). The test cells are also incubated with control group AB serum, which should give a negative result to exclude non-specific reactions. The DAT on the cells should also be negative. Control D-positive cells should be incubated with the standard sera to confirm their activity. The control cells should be group O CDE/cde (R_1r) to show that the antisera are capable of reacting with heterozygous cells.

Many standard anti-D sera are obtained from individuals whose sera also contain anti-A or anti-B. These unwanted antibodies are absorbed using group A and B Rh negative (dd) cells. In order to check that no anti-A or -B remains, which would give false positive results in group A or B subjects, a control test with group AB Rh negative (dd) cells is also included for each standard antiserum. The various reactions set up for blood grouping are given in Table 14.4.

Antibody screening

An antibody screen on recipient serum is performed by incubating it with group O red cells from two or three individuals, who between them carry all the important red cell antigens. Ideally they should be homozygous for each antigen. These cells are either used as a mixed pool or individually, the latter being more sensitive. An autologous control is also set up using recipient's cells versus recipient's serum to exclude an autoantibody. Alternatively a direct antiglobulin test is done on the recipient's cells.

The recipient's serum is tested against the screening cells by several techniques at 37°C, commonly by the indirect antiglobulin test, an

Table 14.4 Reaction mixtures used in blood grouping

Red cells	Serum	Notes
ABO typing room temperature		
test	anti-A	
test	anti-B	Determine ABO group
test	group O	
known group A		Confirms ABO group by
known group B	patient's	'natural' antibodies,
known group O		detects anti-A₁ in A₂ and A₂B subjects.
Controls with each batch		
known group A	with anti-A,	To check reagents for
known group B	anti-B	activity and false
known group O	group O serum	positives
Rhesus (D) typing 37°C		
test	saline anti-D	
test	albumin or enzyme anti-D	Determine D group
test	IAT with anti-D	For weak D, i.e. Du
test	DAT	For autoantibody, should be negative
test	group AB	For non-specific reaction should be negative
Controls		
CDE/cde (R₁r)	with above sera	Should be positive for activity of sera
Group AB, dd		Should be negative. i.e. no ABO anti-bodies in sera or false positives

IAT = indirect antiglobulin test; DAT = direct antiglobulin test

enzyme method, by the addition of albumin and in saline (see later for details). The use of several methods incorporates the advantages of each. In order to ensure that the procedure used is capable of detecting significant antibody a known serum containing weak anti-D is set up against control CDE/cde (R₁r) and cde/cde (rr) cells, by albumin and enzyme methods. It is also usual to incubate the cells/serum mixture in saline at room temperature. This detects 'cold' antibodies such as anti-A₁, -P₁, M, N and LUª, which, if inactive at 37°C, are clinically insignificant. Some authorities, therefore, dispute the usefulness of this.

Having detected the presence of an antibody it is identified using an extended panel of group O cells, each of which is homozygous for one or more important blood group antigen. An example of a commonly used panel is shown in Table 14.5. The technique used depends on that which detected the antibody during the screening procedure. Controls are set up as above.

If an autoantibody is present it is imperative to exclude the presence of an alloantibody, and the investigation of such cases is described on page 134.

The cross-match

The 'cross-match' is regarded as the last and most important test of compatibility between donor cells and recipient serum. The recipient serum and donor cells are incubated together at 37°C by all techniques. Any donor units giving positive results are rejected. Recently, however, the pre-eminence of the cross-match as a method of excluding significant incompatibility has been challenged. Some would argue that, provided the recipient has been fully grouped and the serum screened by a sensitive technique to detect any red cell antibodies, then the cross-match procedure is of less importance, although few would dispense with it completely. Using homozygous screening cells for antibody detection, however, may pick up antibody that would be missed during cross-matching with a donor who is only heterozygous for the corresponding antigen. Such weak antibodies are rarely of immediate clinical importance but may lead to delayed haemolytic transfusion reactions.

These arguments have led to the adoption of the 'group and screen' policy (Table 5.4). For routine operations and obstetrics the patient's blood is grouped and screened for antibodies rather than being fully cross-matched. If a significant blood group antibody is identified, donor units negative for the antigen are tested for and selected. In most cases, no antibody will be found. If blood does become necessary during the operation, units of the correct group are selected, and a rapid cross-match using the LISS technique is used. The blood can then be released for use within 20 minutes. The cross-match safeguards against the presence of an antibody to a rare antigen absent on the screening cells but present on donor cells. The group and screen policy reduces wastage of donor units that are otherwise repeatedly cross-matched for a series of patients, yet never used.

Table 14.5 A typical red cell panel for identification of blood group antibodies with example of results to be expected in presence of anti-Kell (Courtesy of Ortho Diagnostic Systems)

Cell no.	Donor number	Geno-type	Rh-hr D	C	E	c	e	f	C^w	Kell K	k	Duffy Fy^a	Fy^b	Kidd Jk^a	Jk^b	X-linked Xg^a	Lewis Le^a	Le^b	MNS S	s	M	N	P Luth P_1	Lu^a	Special antigen typing	SRT	S37°	ALB	PAP	AHG
1	11103	$R_1^w R_1$	+	+	O	O	+	O	+	+	+	+	O	+	+	O	+	O	O	+	O	O	+	+	O		–	–	–	–	–
2	21824	R_1R_1	+	+	O	O	+	O	O	O	+	+	+	+	+	+	O	O	+	O	+	O	+	+	O		–	–	W	–	C
3	41089	R_2R_2	+	O	+	+	O	O	O	+	+	+	+	O	+	+	O	O	O	+	+	+	O	O	O		–	–	–	–	–
4	91379	$R_o r$	+	O	O	+	+	+	O	O	+	O	O	+	O	O	O	+	O	+	+	+	+	+	+	V+VS+	–	–	–	–	–
5	61089	r'r	O	+	O	+	+	+	O	O	+	+	+	+	+	O	O	+	O	+	+	+	O	O	O		–	–	–	–	–
6	71072	r"r	O	O	+	+	+	+	O	O	+	+	O	O	+	O	O	O	+	O	O	+	$+^s$	O	U+w	–	–	–	–	–
7	81892	rr	O	O	O	+	+	+	O	+	+	O	O	+	+	+	+	+	O	+	+	O	+	O	W	–	–	–	–	C
8	81745	rr	O	O	O	+	+	+	O	O	+	+	+	+	+	O	O	+	+	+	+	O	+	O		–	–	–	–	–
9	81738	rr	O	O	O	+	+	+	O	O	+	+	+	+	+	O	+	O	+	+	+	+	+	+	Bg(b+)	–	–	–	–	–
10	81517	rr	O	O	O	+	+	+	O	O	+	+	+	+	+	+	O	O	O	O	O	+	O	O		–	–	–	–	–
11	F.573	Cord pool															O	O								Sd(a–)I–	–	–	–	–	–
	Patient cells																													

Key: SRT = Saline room temperature
S37° = Saline at 37°C
ALB = Albumin
PAP = Papain
AHG = Antihuman Globulin
+ = Antigen present
O = Antigen absent
– = No reaction
W = Weak agglutination
C = Complete agglutination

Practical aspects of blood transfusion serology

Identification of red cell antigens depends on their reactions with antibodies of known specificity while identification of antibodies depends on their reaction with red cells of known antigenicity. Therefore it is essential to include negative controls to exclude non-specific reactions and positive controls to confirm the reagents' activity. Details of the controls needed were given in the previous section. For manual techniques tests are done in test-tubes, usually small 'precipitin' tubes. For anti-human globulin tests larger volume tubes are used to facilitate washing.

Saline tests

The serum (standard or unknown) is added to the test-tube first, and its presence checked before addition of the red cells. Neat serum is used in most cases, but the standard sera for ABO typing are diluted 1:1 in normal saline to inhibit rouleaux formation. Red cells are suspended in normal saline, as a 3% suspension, as judged by eye. These volumes are delivered using a Pasteur pipette which must be rinsed four times in clean saline between different reagents.

Enzyme tests

For tests involving enzymes, the red cells can be pre-incubated with the enzyme or more simply an equal volume of enzyme is added to the serum before the addition of the red cells. The serum and enzyme must not be left standing for longer than five minutes and the red cells are carefully layered on without mixing. Red cells then fall through the enzyme before reaching the serum. The incubation is done at 37°C for one hour and the results are read microscopically.

Indirect antiglobulin test

For the standard indirect antiglobulin test (IAT) a 3% suspension of red cells is added to serum at a ratio of 1:1. They are mixed, incubated at 37°C for one hour and then washed four times in normal saline. High centrifugal forces are permissible at this stage. The final cell button is resuspended and an equal volume of working strength anti-human globulin (AHG) is added. They are incubated for one minute at room temperature, and centrifuged slowly at 1,000 rpm for two minutes.

The resulting cell button is examined by eye for agglutination; negative results are checked microscopically.

A modification, the 'albumin Coombs" method, involves the addition of albumin to the initial incubation phase, which shortens the test. Four volumes of serum are mixed with one volume of 5% red cells. Three volumes of 30% albumin are added, and the mixture incubated for 20–30 minutes at 37°C. The test is then completed as above.

Low ionic strength saline (LISS)

The use of red cells suspended in low-ionic-strength-saline (LISS) allows incubation times for all techniques to be shortened to ten minutes. LISS has a molarity of 0.33, which is critical to its efficiency. The pH should be 6.7 and contamination should be avoided, sealed containers are therefore used.

The red cells are made up to a 3% suspension in LISS. They are added to an equal volume of serum, and because the final ionic strength is critical the volumes must be accurately dispensed. For enzyme and albumin techniques an equal volume of reagent is used. However, LISS suspended red cells are most often used for antiglobulin tests. The AHG used must not have excessive antiglobulin or anticomplement activity because LISS suspended cells tend to acquire complement from the serum. During the cell washing phase normal saline is used. Techniques employing LISS are very sensitive and, if used correctly, false positives are rare. Recently commercial LISS 'additives' have been introduced. These usually contain a preservative and albumin, and are designed to produce a low ionic strength mixture when added to normal-saline suspended red cells. They may cause slightly greater dilution of test serum (antibody) and are more expensive in use than standard LISS reagents.

Incubation and results

For tests to assign ABO groups or identify 'cold' antibodies incubation is done at room temperature for one and a half hours. Most other tests require 37°C incubation. A water bath allows the temperature to be achieved rapidly, but air incubators are more convenient. Test-tube racks made of material with insulating properties (wood/rubber) should be avoided.

Results are read microscopically and scored according to Table 14.6. Control results should always be read first. AHG test results are read

Table 14.6 Scoring of results of agglutination

C (complete)	Single mass of agglutinated cells visible by naked eye
+++	Large separate masses of agglutinated cells visible
++	Small agglutinates just visible on the slide before micros-cope examination
+	Granular appearance on slide shown to be large clumps of 20+ cells on microscopy
(+)	Clumps of 12–20 cells visible only on microscopy
W (weak)	Clumps of 4–12 cells visible only by microscopy
? or 'sticky'	Cells tend to form groups of 2 or 3 sticking together
0	Negative, all cells evenly distributed on microscopy

N.B. In albumin cells may form loose aggregates, but they are not firm agglutinates; if the slide is rolled, peripheral cells readily detach. This is a negative result.

macroscopically, but negatives are checked microscopically. To exclude false negatives, due to incomplete washing, known strongly sensitized washed red cells are added to negative tubes. These are recentrifuged at 1,000 rpm and should give a positive result. A negative result means that the AHG has been inactivated by contaminating serum.

Emergency procedures

In an emergency blood may have to be given more rapidly than the full grouping, screening and cross-matching procedures allow. In the most urgent situations of blood loss, group O rhesus negative blood, which has been screened for high titre ABO antibodies, can be used. The group of this blood is checked before issue. Alternatively the ABO and rhesus (D) group can be determined using strong saline antisera, especially anti-D. Such antisera are available commercially. Blood of the same ABO and rhesus group (checked before issue) can then be issued uncross-matched.

In the less urgent situation the group is determined as above and the cross-match is set up using LISS-suspended red cells at 37°C with the incubation time cut down to 15 minutes. In this way blood can be ready from scratch in 25 to 30 minutes. While the emergency cross-match is incubating the full grouping and cross-matching procedures are initiated.

Other techniques in the blood transfusion laboratory

Preparation of an eluate

Antibody specifically attached to red cells can be eluted and tested against a panel of red cells in order to identify it. This is useful for the investigation of autoimmune haemolytic anaemia, haemolytic disease of the newborn and some haemolytic transfusion reactions. The final proof that an antibody found in the subject's serum is responsible for haemolysis is its elution from the red cells. The investigation of autoimmune haemolysis is discussed on page 131.

Elution is also used to remove antibodies from red cells, for example in cases of autoimmune haemolysis, in order to allow grouping and cross-matching tests to be carried out on the red cells. For this purpose a method which leaves the red cells intact must be chosen.

Ether method for antibody elution

The sensitized red cells are washed four times in normal saline to remove non-specific contaminating antibody. An aliquot of the final wash solution is retained. Glass tubes must be used. To the packed cells an equal volume of saline is added. Two volumes of diethylether are added to this mixture, the tube is tightly stoppered and contents mixed. The stopper is loosened, and the tube placed in 37°C water bath for 30 minutes. The contents are agitated at intervals. The final mixture is centrifuged at 3,000 rpm for 10 minutes. Three layers result. At the bottom is the haemoglobin stained eluate, separated by a layer of red cell stroma from the ether at the top. The unwanted ether and red cell stroma are removed, the eluate should be placed in a water bath at 37°C for 15 minutes to drive off any traces of ether.

On subsequent testing of the eluate, the aliquot of saline from the final cell wash is used as a control. It should not contain any antibody activity, which confirms that any activity in the eluate is due to antibody specifically attached to the red cell.

Heat elution techniques

Sensitized red cells are washed and packed as above, and an aliquot of the final wash solution is retained as a control. An equal volume of saline is added to the packed cells. The mixture is incubated in a water bath at 56°C for 10 minutes, with repeated shaking and is then immediately centrifuged. The haemoglobin stained supernatent contains the eluted antibody.

By reducing the incubation time to three to five minutes the red cells are left intact but most of the antibody is eluted. This method is useful for producing intact red cells eluted free of autoantibody to use in further tests during investigation of autoimmune haemolytic anaemia. Such red cells can be used to absorb the patient's serum, when the autoantibody should be removed, leaving behind any alloantibody, whose presence must be excluded if blood transfusion is contemplated (page 133).

The ZZAP elution technique

In this the washed red cells are incubated in 0.1M dithiothreitol containing 0.1% papain at pH 6.5 at 37°C for 30 minutes. The antibody is eluted and the cells are enzyme treated at the same time. The treatment may have to be repeated if the DAT remains positive. Such cells can be used for autoadsorption, but the antibody in the eluate is partly degraded by the papain present. The Kell antigens on the red cells are also destroyed.

Adsorption of antibodies

Autoadsorption for removal of autoantibodies

Patient's red cells are washed four times and packed. An equal volume of saline is added. The mixture is incubated at 56°C for three minutes to elute any bound antibody. After centrifugation the eluate is removed. The cells are retained and washed three times. The cells are suspended at 50% concentration in saline and an equal volume of papain is added. They are then incubated at 37°C for 15 minutes, washed twice and packed. These papainized cells are used to absorb an equal volume of the patient's serum at 37°C for 30 minutes. After centrifugation the serum is removed. The adsorption procedure should then be repeated.

The adsorbed serum should now contain no *autoantibody* and antibody screening (page 213) should detect any alloantibody present. If the autoantibody is still present further adsorption of the serum will be necessary. The ZZAP technique is also used to remove antibodies from cells.

Differential adsorption technique

As an alternative to the autoadsorption technique the differential adsorption technique can be used. Here the serum containing the autoantibody is adsorbed with red cells lacking the antigens to the antibody being sought, but carrying the antigen to which the patient has an autoantibody. As described on page 134 this usually means that Kell negative JK^a negative JK^b and Fy^a negative cells are used for the adsorption. They are papainized and used as above.

Adsorption and elution to produce pure standard antisera

In some cases adsorption of specific antibody by standard red cells is a useful way of purifying it. For example, in the rare phenomenon of polyagglutinability, the subject's red cells are agglutinated by almost all typing sera, making grouping impossible. This is usually the result of bacterial infection. Bacterial enzymes digest and alter blood group antigens to produce an antigen known as 'T'. Unfortunately almost all normal individuals have anti-T activity, therefore all grouping sera contain it. If the grouping serum is incubated with cells positive for its own antigen, they can be washed and the antibody (free of anti-T) can be eluted and used to type the patient's cells.

Antibody titre measurement

Having identified an antibody it may be necessary to assess its strength. This is usually a semiquantitative analysis expressed as the reciprocal of the weakest dilution that will cause weak agglutination with standard homozygous red cells. This is called the titre. Knowledge of the titre of an antibody is of great importance in the management of pregnancy in a woman sensitized to fetal red cell antigens (page 155).

The technique chosen to measure an antibody titre depends on that which gave positive results during antibody identification tests, for example, to measure the titre of an anti-Kell antibody the AHG method would be chosen, but to measure anti-D an enzyme technique might be selected. In some cases the titre is measured by all the available techniques and compared.

Master dilutions of the serum to be tested are made. The simplest method is the 'doubling dilutions' technique. An equal volume of diluent (normal saline) is placed in all but the first tube in the row. Neat serum is placed in this. To the second tube in the row a volume of serum equal to the diluent is added and mixed to produce a final dilution of 1:2. Half the volume is then transferred to the third tube and mixed with the diluent present to produce a final dilution of 1:4. The process is repeated and half the volume in the final tube is discarded.

For manual techniques a Pasteur pipette is used. The mixing must be thorough and volumes are measured in drops or by marking the pipette to make sure equal volumes are always drawn up.

The appropriate red cells, at 3% or 5% suspension according to the test being used, are added to each tube in a volume equal to that of the diluted serum. Thus in the first tube neat serum and cells are present; in the second 1:2 diluted serum and cells, etc. This actually reduces the final dilution of serum in each tube by half, but it is convention to express the titre as the reciprocal of the strength of the initial serum dilution in which weak agglutination occurs. Thus if weak agglutination ocurs in the third tube the titre is expressed as 4.

Screening and testing for cold agglutinins

Since all normal sera will show some auto cold agglutinin activity at 4°C it is necessary to test the titre of cold antibody present to show that its presence is abnormally high. It is usual to use doubling dilutions of patient's serum and to set up four replicates.

To each series of dilutions a 2% suspension of red cells is added as follows:

1 Normal pooled group O adult cells (I+).
2 Normal pooled group O cord blood cells (i+).
3 Enzyme treated group O cells.
4 Patient's own red cells separated at 37°C.

The tubes are incubated at 4°C and the results read microscopically using warmed slides.

The normal titre of cold agglutinins is 1 in 32 at 4°C with adult cells, 0–8 at 4°C with cord cells and 1 in 64 with enzyme treated cells. If the titres are higher, significant cold agglutinins are present, and if they are also present in the autocontrol to a similar titre the agglutinin is probably an autoagglutinin.

The thermal amplitude of a cold agglutinin can be assessed by placing ten drops of patient's serum separated at 37°C into three test tubes at 37°C. To the first tube one drop of 50% warmed adult red cells is added, to the second tube one drop of 50% warmed cord red cells and to the third tube one drop of 50% warmed patient's red cells.

The mixtures are incubated for one hour at 37°C, and then transferred to a beaker of water containing a thermometer initially at 37°C. The temperature is allowed to fall, and at 1°C intervals the tubes are inspected for agglutination. Thus the highest temperature at which the antibody is active can be found.

The Donath-Landsteiner test

The IgG cold haemolysins of paroxysmal cold haemoglobinuria are screened for as follows. The patient's blood is collected at 37°C into two tubes, one is placed immediately into a 37°C water bath. The second is placed in ice and kept at 0°C for one hour, after which it is also incubated at 37°C. The tubes are then examined for haemolysis. If the Donath-Lansteiner antibody is present, haemoglobin will be seen in the tube which had been pre-cooled, while that kept at 37°C shows no lysis (control tube). Serum from the non-haemolysed specimen can be added to a 50% suspension of standard P-positive red cells, at a volume of 9:1. The mixture is cooled on ice for one hour, incubated at 37°C for 30 minutes and then centrifuged. Visible lysis confirms that the IgG, anti-P Donath Landsteiner antibody was present in the serum. A control tube kept at 37°C should show no lysis. Occasionally it is necessary to add a small amount of normal serum to the test to supply complement if the patient has recently had a severe attack.

Neutralization of IgM antibody using dithiothreitol (DTT)

During investigation of ABO haemolytic disease of the newborn and some autoimmune disorders, it is sometimes useful to know whether the antibody is IgG or IgM. One method of doing this is to inactivate any IgM present using dithiothreitol which disrupts the interchain di-sulphide bonds of IgM forming inactive 7S subunits. The Fc portion of the molecule is still intact and can be detected using anti-IgM-heavy chain.

Equal volumes of undiluted serum and 0.01M DTT (in phosphate buffer pH 7.4) are incubated for 30 minutes at 37°C. A control incubation of serum plus buffer is also set up. The treated serum and control are then titrated against appropriate red cells in the usual way. If the antibody was IgM, none will be present in the DTT treated serum, but activity will be present in the control serum. If the antibody was IgG, activity will be present in the DTT treated and control sera.

Control cells for specific antiglobulin tests

In some cases it is important to know whether red cells are coated with complement only, and with which component, or whether cells are coated with IgG or IgM. For example such knowledge is useful in diagnosis of autoimmune haemolytic anaemias (page 132). In order to ensure that the antiglobulin reagent used will detect the component sought it is necessary to use control coated red cells.

IgG

To sensitize cells with IgG one volume of 50% group O D positive cells is incubated with ten volumes of incomplete anti-D for one hour. The cells are then washed four times. They will be agglutinated by AHG containing anti-human IgG antibody.

IgM

Serum known to contain lytic IgM anti-Le^a is treated with EDTA at pH 7.0 at a ratio of 10:1. This prevents complement binding. One volume of a 50% suspension of Le^a positive group O cells is then incubated with ten volumes of this serum for one hour at 37°C. The washed red cells are IgM coated.

Complement

C4 coated red cells are produced by adding a 50% suspension of group O cells to nine volumes of serum known to contain an incomplete cold antibody. The mixture is placed in ice for two hours and washed four times in saline at 37°C. The cells will be coated with C4 only.

C4, C3b and C3d can be attached to group O red cells by suspending them in LISS and incubating at 37°C for 15 minutes. The LISS used is 60 g/litre sucrose in 0.02M NaCl. The cells are washed four times in normal saline. C3d alone will remain on the red cells of a patient with known cold agglutinin disease if they are washed four times in saline at 37°C.

Automation of blood group serology

There are two major types of automatic blood grouping machines.

Both rely on the fact that red cell agglutinates sediment more rapidly than unagglutinated red cells.

The continuous flow auto-analyser (for example the Technicon Auto-Analyser) uses peristaltic pumps to draw up and mix samples and reagents which move into a manifold at the desired temperature where antibody/antigen interaction occurs. Successive samples and reagents are separated by air bubbles in the system of tubing. Agglutination is enhanced by the use of rouleaux-producing agents such as polyvinyl-pyrrolidone (PVP) and the enzyme bromelin, or polybrene and low ionic strength media. Having passed through the reaction chamber, the rouleaux are dispersed by the injection of saline so that only true agglutinates remain. The mixture of agglutinates and non-agglutinated cells then passes through settling coils and the sedimented agglutinates are drawn off. The remaining unagglutinated cells then pass through a continuous flow photometer at 850 nm.

The results are recorded continuously. The baseline represents the haemoglobin concentration when there is no reaction and 100% of cells remain unagglutinated, the depth of fall of absorbance from this level is proportional to the number cells agglutinated, that is to the strength of antibody–antigen reaction.

With known red cells the presence of specific antibody can be detected in test sera, or using standard antisera the blood group of red cell samples can be determined. For each standard reagent a separate channel is needed. Where international standards are available antibody can be accurately quantified using such machines (for example anti-D). Fig. 14.2 shows a single channel auto-analyser.

The 'Groupmatic' automated blood grouping system also relies on the fact that agglutinates settle more rapidly than unagglutinated cells. Here the red cells and serum are mixed in a shallow concave translucent well. If agglutination occurs, then the majority of red cells fall to the centre of the well. If no agglutination occurs, the red cells are spread evenly across the bottom of the well. The difference in transmission of a beam of light through the centre of the well and through the edge is measured, and the greater the difference the stronger the antibody–antigen reaction. The machine can be used for antibody identification or red cell grouping.

The Groupmatic and Technicon auto-analysers are expensive machines with high running costs. However, the increasing use of transparent plastic microwell plates instead of test-tubes in blood transfusion laboratories has led to the development of a technique for automatic reading of results. Appropriate grouping sera and test cells are

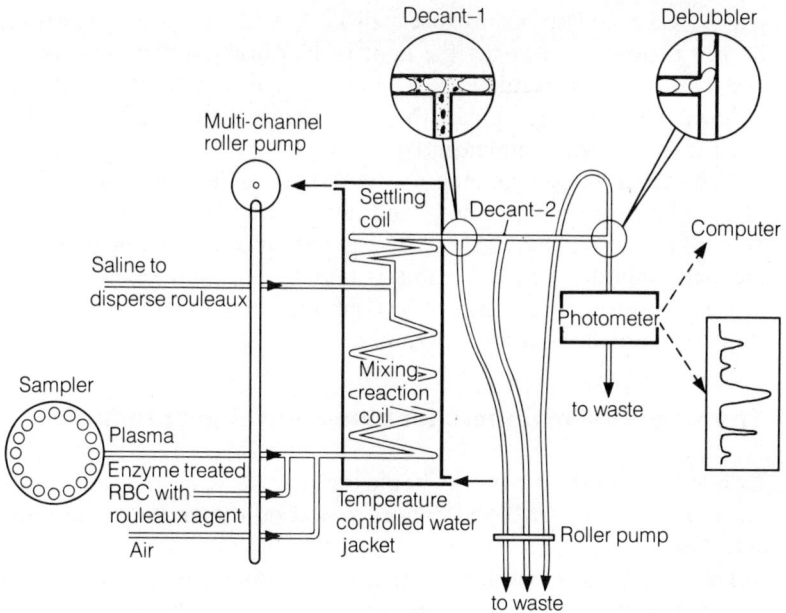

Fig. 14.2 Diagrammatic representation of automated antibody screening using the Technicon Autogrouper-16C. The samples are fed into the machine at the sampler, where a barcode reader identifies each specimen for use in the computer output. The machine has 16 channels and can be set up for routine blood grouping or other serological investigations.

After the reagents have been mixed with the sample, antigen/antibody reaction takes place at the appropriate temperature, the length of incubation being determined by the length of the reaction coil; any rouleaux are then dispersed with saline. The agglutinates settle out in the settling coil and are decanted off. The number of cells remaining in suspension is then determined in a photometer. The results are either analysed by computer or from the recorder tracing.

mixed and allowed to react in the wells. In 'positive' wells a tight dark clump of agglutinated cells with an irregular edge can be seen with the naked eye. In 'negative' wells a diffuse, even distribution of dispersed cells is seen. The results can be read automatically on a machine such as the Dynatech MR600 reader which measures the absorbance of a beam of light passed through the microplate contents. The absorbance of the supernatants is used to assess whether a reaction has taken place. If red cells remain evenly suspended (a negative result), then the absorbance will be high. If the red cells have agglutinated, the supernatant will be clear and so absorbance will be low. To ensure agglutinates do not themselves obstruct the light path (causing a high absorbance and false negative result), the reader is tilted at 17° so agglutinates sediment clear of the light path. A computer is used to convert the readings into positive and negative results.

Automated blood grouping and serology enables hundreds of samples to be processed per hour and allows accurate quantification of antibodies. Sensitivity of the test is greatly increased compared with manual methods; sometimes this is unhelpful as antibodies detected at very low levels which cannot be confirmed by sensitive manual techniques are usually clinically insignificant.

The selection of donors for blood and blood products

Donors of blood or plasma should be over 18 years old and under 60. However, regular blood donors may continue to donate until the age of 65.

The hazards of blood donation in the previously normal individual are few but include syncope, very rarely cardiac arrhythmia and haematoma or infection at the venepuncture site. The risks of plasmapheresis or cell separation for donors are outlined in Chapter 12.

Exclusion to prevent donor morbidity

Individuals should be excluded from donation if the following are found:

1 Weight under 50 kg.
2 Anaemia; arrangements for further investigations should be made.
3 Previous donation less than 16 weeks previously; individuals should not donate blood more than twice yearly. Plasmapheresis may be done more frequently.
4 If the donor's occupation is hazardous, for example, working at height, there must be time for recovery (several hours) before he intends to resume such activity; he should not ride a motorcycle shortly after donation.
5 History of minor surgery or trauma within the previous four weeks, or major surgery or trauma within the previous six months.
6 History of cardiovascular disease, epilepsy or diabetes, requiring insulin or drugs for their control; for all these patients a sudden exacerbation may follow blood donation.

7 History of gastrectomy; impaired iron absorption will delay recovery from blood donation.

Exclusion to prevent recipient morbidity

The most serious hazard for transfusion recipients apart from transfusion reaction, is blood-transmitted infection.

Donors who have any of the following should not be accepted:

1 Hepatitis. Individuals should be asked to wait one year after an attack of hepatitis before donating blood. If HBsAg is present, they will then be rejected. Under certain circumstances, patients who have had hepatitis B will be reinstated as donors if sensitive tests (page 141) show them to be HBsAg negative and they have over 1 iu/ml of anti-HBsAg antibody in their serum. Individuals who have had acupuncture, ear-piercing or tattooing must wait six months before donating blood.

2 AIDS. Donors who are in high risk groups for transmitting HTLV III such as male homo- and bi-sexuals, drug addicts, natives of Haiti and Central Africa and thier sexual partners are not accepted.

3 Other Viral Infections. Individuals who have active viral infections or who have been vaccinated with live vaccines for measles, mumps, rabies, smallpox or yellow fever must wait one month before donation. After rubella vaccination, three months must elapse before donation. During this time they may, however, usefully give plasma for immune globulin preparation. A donor who has had documented glandular fever should not be accepted until two years after the diagnosis was made.

4 Miscellaneous Infections. Toxoplasmosis patients should not donate blood until one year after the toxoplasma dye test has become negative. Brucellosis and a history of syphilis contraindicate donation. Patients with tuberculosis under treatment, or who are close contacts of active cases should not be accepted.

5 Tropical Diseases. Patients with filariasis, kala azar, trypanosomiasis, leptospirosis or yaws should be disqualified. Any person recently arrived from a tropical area should wait six months before being accepted as a blood donor.

Malaria.
Individuals who have had malaria or who have recently arrived from malarious areas should wait six months before donation, and

then their blood should only be used for production of albumin-containing fractions. However, if over five years have elapsed since arrival from a malarious area and there is no history of an attack, blood may be accepted and used for all purposes.

6   Disorders such as Creutzfeld-Jakob disease or multiple sclerosis may be due to 'slow virus' infections and such patients should not give blood.

7   Other conditions. Haemophiliacs should not become blood donors. Symptomless carriers may donate blood but it should not be used for production of coagulation concentrates.

8   Cancer patients should not be accepted.

Further reading

Dacie, J V, Lewis, S M (1984) Blood groups and laboratory aspects of blood transfusion. In: *Practical Haematology, 6th Edn*. Churchill Livingstone, Edinburgh.

Boorman, K E, Dodd, B E, Lincoln, P J (1977) *Blood Group Serology. Theory techniques, Practical Applications, 5th Edn*. Churchill Livingstone, Edinburgh.

Issitt, P D, Issitt, C H (1977) *Applied Blood Group Serology, 2nd Edn*. Spectra Biologicals, Becton Dickinson and Co.

Muller, A, Garetta, M, Herbert, M (1981) Groupmatic system: overview, history of development and evaluation of use. *Vox Sanguinis* 40, 201–13.

Moore, B P L (1969) Automation in the Blood Transfusion Laboratory. *Canadian Medical Association Journal* 100, 381

Bowley, A R, Gordon, I, Ross, D W (1984) Computer controlled automated reading of blood groups using microplates. *Medical and Laboratory Sciences*, 41, 19–28.

Index